PRINCIPLES OF BRAIN STIMULATION

Principles
of Brain Stimulation

JOHN STANTON YEOMANS

New York   Oxford
OXFORD UNIVERSITY PRESS
1990

Oxford University Press

Oxford   New York   Toronto
Delhi   Bombay   Calcutta   Madras   Karachi
Petaling Jaya   Singapore   Hong Kong   Tokyo
Nairobi   Dar es Salaam   Cape Town
Melbourne   Auckland

and associated companies in
Berlin   Ibadan

Copyright © 1990 Oxford University Press, Inc.

Published by Oxford University Press, Inc.,
200 Madison Avenue, New York, New York 10016

Oxford is a registered trademark of Oxford University Press

Library of Congress Cataloging-in-Publication Data
Yeomans, John Stanton.
Principles of brain stimulation / John Stanton Yeomans.
p. cm. Bibliography: p. Includes index. ISBN 0-19-506138-1
1. Brain stimulation. I. Title.
[DNLM: 1. Brain—Physiology. 2. Electric Stimulation.
WL 300 Y46p] QP388.Y46 1990 152—dc20
DNLM/DLC   for Library of Congress   89-16137

The author gratefully thanks the original publishers
for the use of several previously published figures
and two short quotations. These are individually cited
in the figures and text. Franco Vaccarino provided
the photograph of Figure 4-1.

9 8 7 6 5 4 3 2 1
Printed in the United States of America
on acid-free paper

Preface

Many books have been written on the subject of electrical brain stimulation. I have tried to write a very different book, more neurophysiological and more systematic, that reflects how the field has changed in the last 10 years and points the direction to future changes. In particular, this book emphasizes the axonal basis of brain stimulation. Especially, double-pulse stimulation methods that describe the absolute refractory periods, conduction velocities, and connections of the axons responsible for electrically evoked behaviors are developed thoroughly here for the first time.

Also, I have tried to propose a more standard methodology. (This idea did not please me at first—science must allow the maximum freedom for creativity, and the idea seemed slightly authoritarian.) I've gradually come to believe that the methods of brain stimulation can be derived from fundamental principles. Principles of neural excitation influence the choices of waveform, and temporal and spatial parameters. Principles of psychophysics influence the choices of measurement procedures. Stimulation methods should be chosen that allow the clearest interpretation at the neuronal level, and that allow investigators to compare their stimulation intensities quantitatively. These criteria do not leave much room for freedom, since electrical excitation of neurons is a precise field. This credo did not warm my heart, but I think one must be warmed by the prospect of a better science.

The difficulty of writing a "principles" book is that ideas are rarely completely rigorous, completely generalizable, and easily developed at the same time. Since brain stimulation is practiced by biophysical engineers, motor physiologists, surgeons, and psychologists, I have tried to choose a "middle ground" that would be useful to all these potential readers, and still make a solid introduction to the topic. In several cases, I have oversimplified issues that are developed in more detail in the cited articles. I have often failed to discuss interesting phenomena that do not, for me, clarify more general issues. I can only hope that the need for a systematic introduction to brain stimulation outweighs any shortcomings of this first attempt, and that later versions will benefit from this book. Although chemical stimulation is not discussed, several of the principles are applicable to that burgeoning field.

This text is aimed at the advanced undergraduate or graduate student in neuroscience, although there is some more advanced material for specialists. Chapters 2 and 3 contain fundamentals that must be understood, but readers may then wish to skip to Chapter 6 if they are interested in double-pulse studies. An appreciation of simple mathematical concepts is very helpful.

Many people have helped me think about these problems. Tony Deutsch and Randy Gallistel each advised me with wit about the perils of research, and the joys of double-pulse experiments. Peter Shizgal devised several of the experiments presented in this book and has been a constant source of valuable ideas and encouragement. Bob Hawkins, George Fouriezos, Cathy Bielajew, Theris Miliaressis, Gary Matthews, Peter Milner, and Roy Wise have all been able colleagues and good friends who made technical advances on some of the problems mentioned here. I have been influenced by the work of K. Lucas, H. S. Gasser, W. R. Hess, A. Hodgkin, B. Katz, J. Ranck and H. Asanuma and their colleagues and thank them all, even those who are dead. These beneficent influences must not, however, be blamed for the inadequacies contained herein. I especially apologize for citing my own papers over other excellent work that I am less familiar with.

The book is dedicated to all students of brain stimulation, including my own two Ph.D. students, Ora Kofman and Ed Tehovnik, for whom this book was originally written. My loving wife, Mary-Ellen, and children, Michael, Katie, and Lauren, have endured the time I have spent away from them in this effort as patiently as can be hoped for.

So here it is finally.

Toronto   J.Y.
April 1989

Contents

PRINCIPLES OF BRAIN STIMULATION

1

A Brief History of Brain Stimulation

Hundreds of different responses, from muscle twitches to complex thoughts, can be elicited by brain stimulation. The neural organization of these responses has been studied by mapping brain sites where responses can be evoked. Over the last hundred years, the electrical stimuli, the neural or behavioral responses to those stimuli, and the spatial resolution of the maps have become better defined.

The value of electrical stimulation lies in the prospect of defining the fundamental components of thought, feeling, and action in terms of the activity of neurons. In most cases, however, the neurons and neural pathways whose excitation produces the responses have not yet been determined, although possible anatomical pathways are often known. The most detailed search has involved the stimulation and recording of the motor cortex with microelectrodes, so studies of the motor cortex will be a special focus of this chapter.

THE DISCOVERY OF ELECTRICAL EXCITABILITY

In the 1790s, two Italians had an argument that historians of physics and neurophysiology still delight in. Luigi Galvani found that frog legs twitch when the muscles are placed against two different metal conductors. Galvani believed that this result proved that frog legs have internal electricity.

Alessandro Volta argued that Galvani was wrong, that the metals themselves were producing the electricity. Volta proved that two metals could produce electricity alone without any muscles attached. He piled zinc and silver disks on top of one another in a salt solution and created the first battery (called the *voltaic pile* in the nineteenth century). Volta argued that the frogs legs in Galvani's experiment simply provided the salt solution needed by the metals to produce electricity.

If that were the end of the story, neurophysiologists would not enjoy it as much as physicists. Galvani persisted and proved that isolated muscles contracted without metals being present. For example, the same twitch occurred when a cut nerve touched the muscle. Therefore, the cut nerve might be carrying an electrical signal also. The next hundred years of neurophysiology involved delivering various electrical stimuli (measured by *galvanometers* and *voltmeters*) to isolated nerves and muscles, and measuring the effect by the size of the muscle twitch. In the end, both Galvani and his frog "nerve-muscle preparation" were vindicated.

Mechanism and the nerve-muscle preparation

The greatest early advances in understanding nerve excitability were made in Germany between 1835 and 1855 by students of Johannes Müller. These students believed that the principles of life can be understood by application of the principles of physics, in other words, that living organisms are just complicated electrochemical mechanisms. This idea was abhorrent to Müller and most other biologists, who called themselves "vitalists," and believed that special vital forces beyond ordinary physics are necessary to keep tissue alive and mobile.

The "mechanists" around Müller favored Galvani's nerve-muscle preparation, because the lifelike twitches of muscles were evoked by measurable electrical forces. The first breakthrough for the mechanists came when Emil DuBois-Reymond showed that there is indeed an electrical charge inside the nerve that carries the "action potential," thereby restoring Galvani's work to prominence. Then, Hermann von Helmholtz (1850) measured the conduction velocity of the action potential along the nerve. The latency of the muscle response was found to be shorter when stimulating the nerve near the muscle than when stimulating the nerve at a long distance from the muscle. Helmholtz then showed that the same was true of human leg nerves. The measured conduction velocities in nerves were, to the astonishment of all, less than a millionth of the velocity of electrical conduction in wires, however.

By presenting two stimuli at a single point, Helmholtz observed what was later called the neural refractory period (Gallistel, 1973). That is, the second stimulus failed to produce a larger twitch when the two stimuli were too close together. Helmholtz did not continue the two-stimulus experiments, and so did not get credit for discovering the neural refractory period, which was rediscovered by Gotch and Burch (1899).

Measuring devices

It is hard for students familiar with oscilloscopes, transistors, and computers to appreciate the difficulty of those early experiments. The responses were crudely measured by attaching wires to the muscle and connecting the wires to pens.

Accurate timing devices were not available in the nineteenth century (Geddes, 1984). To improve his measure of the conduction velocity of nerve, Helmholtz invented a timer for his stimulator based on the pendulum (Figure 1-1). The pendulum was dropped rapidly past two closely spaced contacts. When the pendulum touched the first contact, the current from the battery started. The second contact could be used to stop the current to form a pulse stimulus, or to start a second short-duration stimulus. The time between stimuli was determined by the length of the pendulum and the distance (d) between contacts. A

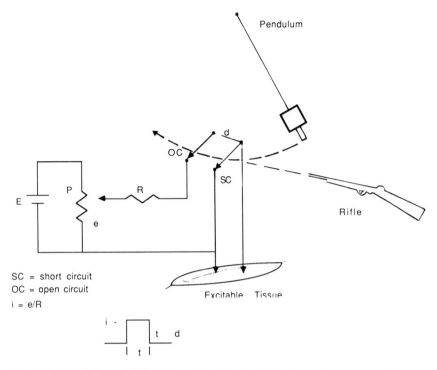

Figure 1-1. Helmholtz' pendulum stimulator (after Geddes, 1984). A pendulum was dropped through two switches, thereby connecting and then disconnecting the battery. This produced a pulse-shaped stimulus. To obtain shorter pulse durations, Weiss (1901) substituted a rifle for the pendulum. The bullet cut the wires.

similar pendulum device (built by Lucas) was still being used in the 1930s by Hodgkin in his first experiments (Hodgkin, 1983).

Helmholtz's pendulum was accurate to only about a millisecond, so faster devices were needed by the end of the century. Weiss (1901) used a high-power rifle to break two wires: breaking the first wire connected the battery; breaking the second wire disconnected the battery. The duration of the stimulus was varied by altering the distance between the wires. This device allowed Weiss and later the Lapicques in France to study the effects of short-duration stimuli, and thereby study the strength–duration curve (Geddes, 1984).

Electrical properties of nerve

By the early twentieth century, peripheral nerve physiologists (such as Lucas, Adrian, and Kato) had studied the main properties of nerve excitability and conductivity (Katz, 1939). Erlanger and Gasser (1937) were the first to use an oscilloscope to record the latency of action potentials. Since the oscilloscope allowed measurements with over a million times more precision than pen recorders, Erlanger and Gasser were able to show the separate latencies of the fast and slow fibers in nerve bundles.

By the turn of the century, however, it was already clear that the principles of nerve excitability by themselves would not be adequate to understand the central nervous system. Sherrington's (1906) studies of spinal reflexes showed that new principles of summation and inhibition govern the functional connections between spinal cells. He named these functional connections *synapses*. The brain was expected to be much more complex.

BRAIN MAPS

From 1870 to 1950, the most effective method of studying brain function was electrical stimulation. Electrical stimulation effects were more localized and more reversible than were lesion effects, and were therefore more easily mapped. Recording brain activity became possible only when amplifiers became available in the 1920s, and recording maps were still crude until single-unit microelectrode recording began in the 1950s.

Maps of motor cortex

The first successful electrical mapping study of the brain was accomplished by Theodor Fritsch. Fritsch was a physician during the Prusso-Danish War of 1864, who noticed, while dressing head wounds near the battlefield, that touching the cerebral cortex produced muscle twitches on the opposite side of the body. When he returned home, Fritsch tested this idea by applying current from a battery to the surface of a dog's cortex. This stimulation produced four different motor responses (neck, forelimb, face, and hindlimb movements) in four different cortical regions (Fritsch & Hitzig, 1870). Stimulating a single site repeatedly resulted in declining responsiveness, probably due to lesioning. By lowering insulated insect pins into the cortex and subcortex, Fritsch and Hitzig were able to prove that the response was evoked in the cortex itself.

Shortly thereafter, David Ferrier (1876, 1886) mapped the cortex of several species. His stimulator was an induction coil that delivered short-duration stimuli of balanced charge. This stimulator allowed Ferrier to stimulate cortical areas over and over again for hours without deterioration of the response. Calibration was still crude, however. Ferrier recommended that an ideal brain stimulus is one that just elicits a taste sensation when applied to the tongue. His tongue was apparently a better judge of effective intensity than the galvanometer readings.

Ferrier showed that the motor cortex in each of these species has a complete body map, often with the body upside down (feet up, head down). His maps of the rhesus monkey and dog are shown in Figure 1-2. Many areas of the cortex were found to be "silent"; that is, no response to stimulation was observed.

In subsequent decades, hundreds of such maps were made of motor cortex in dozens of species from rat to chimpanzee, and eventually of human. It was

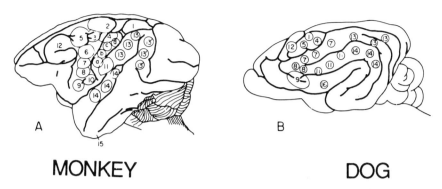

MONKEY   DOG

Figure 1-2. Ferrier's (1886) maps of the motor cortex of the rhesus monkey and dog. The circled numbers show regions where particular movements were evoked: 1–3, leg movements; 4–6, arm (forepaw) and hand movements; 7–11, mouth movements; 12–14, eye and head movements; 15, nostril movements.

discovered that the size of the cortical regions varies considerably between species. The size is not determined by the absolute size of each body part, but appears to be related to the use and sensitivity of each body part. In humans, therefore, the cortical areas for the digits, tongue, and lips are especially large (Penfield & Jasper, 1954) (Figure 1-3).

Woolsey (1958) compared the size of motor areas to somatosensory areas. He mapped the sensory areas by recording electrical potentials in the cortex evoked by touching the body surface. In all animals, he found a large sensory map opposite to (and normally posterior to) the large motor map; again the sizes of different body regions varied in different species (Figure 1-4). For example, Woolsey found that touching the whiskers (vibrissae) of rats activates a huge area (almost half) of the somatosensory cortex. In sheep, who eat grass most of the day, the mouth region is larger than the rest of the entire body. In spider monkeys, with prehensile tails, the tail region is very large.

Maps of deep brain sites

Many early investigators, including Ferrier and Fritsch and Hitzig, stimulated the deep brain with long electrodes that were covered with insulating varnish except at their tips. Many responses similar to those activated by stimulation of the cortex were observed. Deep brain sites were harder to hit accurately because they could not be seen from the surface, while surface sites could be identified relative to visible surface landmarks such as blood vessels or sulci.

Near the turn of the century, Horsley and Clark devised a frame, which they called a *stereotaxic instrument,* for holding the head in a fixed position. Attached to the frame were bars that could be moved in medial–lateral, anterior–posterior, or dorsal–ventral directions. Electrodes could be attached to the movable bars to place lesioning or stimulating electrodes accurately into any small structure deep within the brain. Brain atlases for several species were

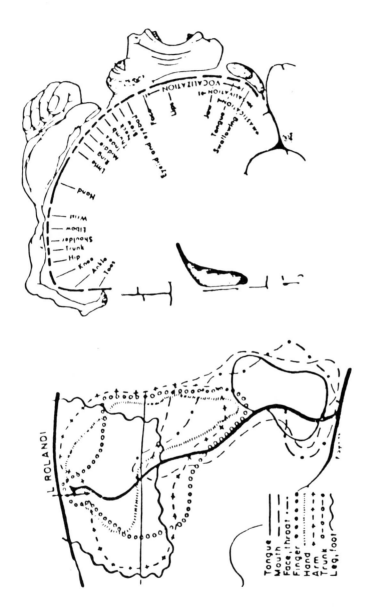

HUMAN

Figure 1-3. Penfield's maps of the human sensory and motor cortex (Penfield & Jasper, 1954). Left, lateral view; right, coronal view, with homunculus.

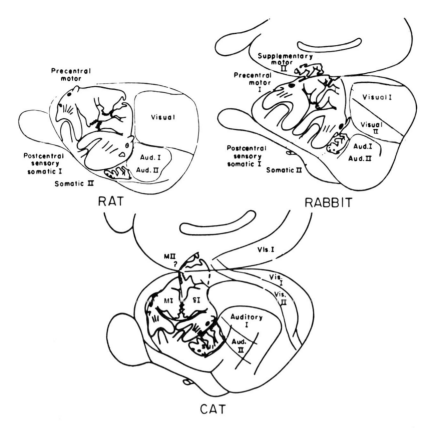

Figure 1-4. Woolsey's (1958) maps of the rat, rabbit, and cat sensory and motor cortex. These maps and ''animunculi'' are schematic summaries of detailed point-by-point tests.

later published, so that the stereotaxic coordinates of each deep brain structure could be identified relative to the position of the skull (Figure 1-5).

Walter Rudolf Hess developed methods in the 1920s and 1930s for attaching electrodes to the skull with small screws and denture cement (Hess, 1957). These methods allowed electrical stimulation of deep brain regions in freely behaving animals over long periods of time (Figure 1-6). Hess took moving pictures of cats stimulated via electrodes placed in many regions of the diencephalon and midbrain. Stimulation of some sites evoked hissing in his cats, while stimulation of other sites evoked purring. In a few sites, stimulation elicited autonomic responses, such as urination or sexual responses, while grooming, feeding, or drinking responses were observed in others. Even these complex behaviors could be turned on and off with pushbutton control.

The responses most commonly observed by Hess were eye and head movements similar to those that Ferrier observed stimulating the frontal eye fields of the monkey cortex. Stimulation evoked movements of both eyes together, most often in the horizontal direction. The eye movements were often immediately

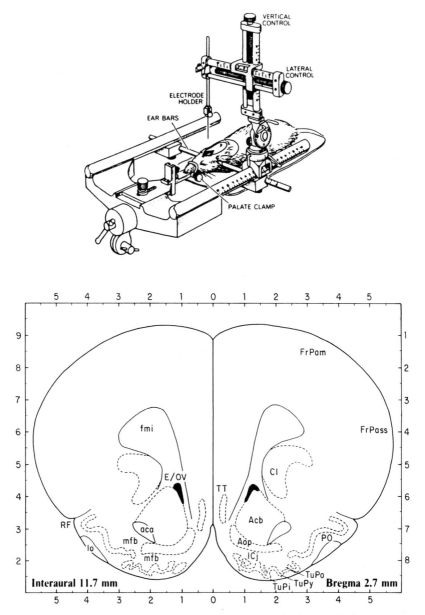

Figure 1-5. Above, a stereotaxic instrument for placing electrodes into deep brain structures. The electrode can be moved independently in vertical, lateral, and anterior directions. Below, one page of a stereotaxic atlas showing a coronal section of the rat brain 11.7 mm anterior to the ear bars (Paxinos & Watson, 1982). Scales are in mm from skull landmarks.

followed by lateral head movements, then by body movements strong enough so that the cat turned completely around (Figure 1-6). These were not just twitches in local muscle groups, but were organized orientation responses of the whole body, as if the cat were turning around to respond to something behind.

Hundreds of behavioral responses evoked by brain stimulation have since been cataloged. Most heavily referenced are limb movements, eye movements, feeding and drinking responses, attack and aversive responses, pain inhibition, and "self-stimulation" (Valenstein, 1973). Many studies of autonomic responses, nesting and grooming responses, vocalizations, forward locomotion, lateral head and body movements, and posture changes have been reported.

Human brain stimulation

The most dramatic studies of electrical stimulation have been performed on human patients undergoing brain surgery for life-threatening brain diseases, such as tumors, or scars leading to epileptic seizures (Penfield & Jasper, 1954) (Figure 1-7). The stimulation has the therapeutic value of helping the surgeon decide which functional brain areas to remove and which to spare during surgery. Only local anesthesia of the region around the incision is given so that these patients are awake and can report the sensations evoked by the electrical stimulation. The poor patient must sit quietly and answer questions precisely to aid the doctor in saving his or her life and in sparing precious brain tissue.

Stimulation of the human motor cortex evokes muscle twitches much like those observed in animals. The patients report that these movements cannot be stopped or controlled voluntarily during the stimulation. Stimulation of the auditory or visual cortex evokes sensations of simple tones or lights, respectively.

In cortical areas that are silent to stimulation in animals, complex feelings, experiences, or urges are reported during stimulation. Stimulation of the temporal lobe (or perhaps the underlying hippocampus) evokes reports of "flashbacks"; that is, experiences in the patient's past (Penfield & Jasper, 1954; Halgren, 1982). Stimulation of limbic areas results in sensations of pain, discomfort, anxiety, or, by contrast, relaxation, pleasure, or pain inhibition (Mark & Ervin, 1970; Iacono & Nashold, 1982; Tasker et al., 1982). Stimulation of cortical speech areas results in very specific verbal deficits, such as losses in word finding, in word order (syntax), or in grammar (Ojemann, 1982).

Wilder Penfield became the most important popularizer of the accomplishments of neurosurgery and of human brain stimulation. His many scientific and autobiographical books dramatize the neurosurgical arena and the quest for understanding of the brain. Penfield wrote freely about the "mystery of mind" and the "landscapes of thought," phrases that filled students with wonder, but sometimes aroused skepticism in fellow scientists. For example, here is his description of temporal lobe stimulation:

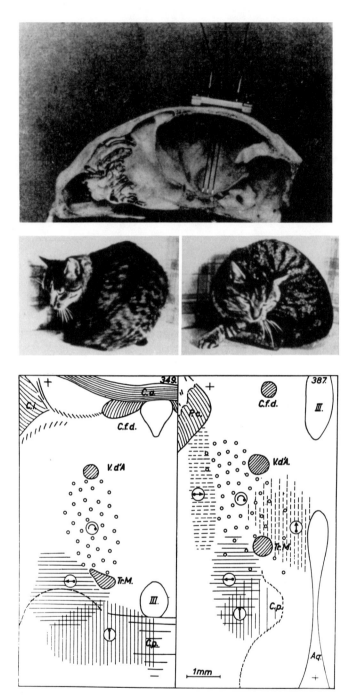

Figure 1-6. Top photograph shows Hess' (1957) device for delivering depth stimulation, shown on a cat skull that has been sectioned at the midline. The connector is mounted to the skull chronically with small screws, and the external wires are attached before each test. Middle photographs show two frames of Hess' moving pictures of an ipsilateral movement evoked by diencephalic stimulation. Below, coronal sections show where ipsilateral movements (horizontal lines and left arrow), contralateral movements (horizontal broken lines and right arrow), vertical sinking movements (vertical lines and down arrow), vertical raising movements (vertical broken lines and up arrow), and rolling in frontal plane (circles and bent arrow) were evoked. These maps summarize dozens of placements.

The electrode [placed on the temporal lobe] causes the patient to have a psychical experience, like the memory of some past event, and he can describe it as he lies upon the operating table. . . . The experience may seem to the patient to be a dream, rather than an accurate memory. But it is a dream in which familiar places are seen and well-known people speak and act. Such hallucinations, or memories, or dreams continue to unfold slowly while the electrode shield is held in place. They are terminated suddenly when the electrode is withdrawn (Penfield & Jasper, 1954, pp. 142–43).

Electrotherapy

In the nineteenth century, electrical stimulation was tried as a treatment for many disorders. Current was passed through the head to treat psychosis, through the muscles to treat pain, through the chest to treat heart disease, or through the genitals to treat infertility (McNeal, 1977). In most cases, better or safer therapies have become available.

Many of these electrotherapies are still in use, however, in an improved form. Electroshock therapy, the passing of milliampere currents through the head, is still widely used to relieve depression. Stimulation of peripheral nerves, the spinal cord, or the thalamus often relieves chronic pain in patients that do

Figure 1-7. Brain stimulation of human patient undergoing brain surgery (Penfield & Jasper, 1954). Only the exposed brain is seen here. Numbers are placed on each brain site that has been stimulated.

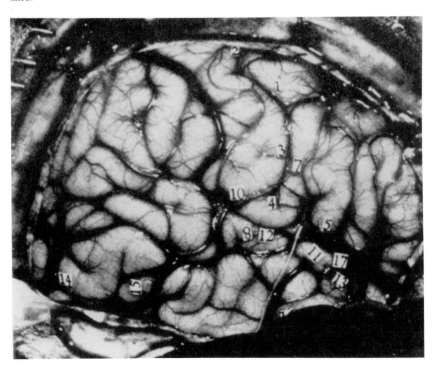

not respond to drug treatments. Stimulation of the cerebellum is used to treat epilepsies, movement disorders, and psychoses (Myklebust et al., 1985). Electrical stimulation across the chest is still the fastest and safest way to restart a heart muscle that has stopped beating. Electrical stimulation of muscles can maintain muscle fitness or occasionally relieve muscle discomfort.

Electricity is even still used to aid fertility. Electrodes placed in the rectum can stimulate autonomic nerves in order to evoke seminal emissions or erections (Brindley, 1981). Although originally used to collect semen in prize bulls, this "electroejaculation" has recently been used by several paraplegics and their wives hoping to overcome infertility. Only one successful live birth has been reported, but several of the wives have been instructed how to use the electrodes on their husbands.

IN PURSUIT OF SINGLE NEURONS

Brain mapping work localizes brain sites where responses can be elicited. It is much harder to determine which neurons within these regions are responsible for producing the responses. The understanding of the neuronal basis of the stimulation-elicited responses awaited the understanding of the electrical properties of single neurons, studied first in peripheral nerves, and later with microelectrodes in the brain.

Single axons

In the early decades of the twentieth century, physiologists proved that electrical responses in peripheral nerve result from exciting many single axons at the same time (Lucas, 1917a; Erlanger & Gasser, 1937). Kato isolated single axons by dissecting frog nerves into the smallest fibers and testing their individual conduction properties. Tasaki (1959) studied the properties of single myelinated axons by stimulating them with microelectrodes at and between the nodes of Ranvier.

The ionic mechanism of the action potential was discovered in the early 1950s. Hodgkin and Huxley (1952) found that squid giant axons are more permeable to sodium ions during the action potential, and that this sodium permeability accounts for the mechanism and shape of the action potential. Similar ionic mechanisms were shown to be responsible for action potentials of mammalian peripheral axons and muscles.

The action potentials found in axons and muscles result from proteins embedded in the cell wall that alter their permeability to sodium when stimulated. When the voltage across the membrane is reduced, these proteins alter their shape and thereby open a channel through the center of the protein through which sodium ions can pass (Hille, 1981), hence the name "voltage-gated sodium channel." The chemical composition of the long chains of amino acids that make up these proteins is now known, amino acid by amino acid, and the three-dimensional folding of these amino acid chains is close to being completely determined (Noda et al., 1986).

The electrical properties of single voltage-gated sodium channels have recently been studied by sucking up a tiny piece of membrane into a smooth-tipped micropipette electrode (Neher & Sakmann, 1976). The action potential results from the simultaneous opening (and then closing) of thousands of voltage-gated sodium channels.

Single brain cells

Microelectrodes were applied to single brain cells in the 1950s to record their activity. Metal microelectrodes were first used to record action potentials from outside cerebral cortex cells (Mountcastle, 1957; Hubel & Wiesel, 1962). One important discovery of single-unit recording was that the cortex is divided up into narrow columns of cells with similar receptive fields. That is, when a microelectrode is passed through the cortex perpendicular to the surface, all cells recorded along the track respond to similar stimuli.

More recently, glass micropipettes have been inserted into single brain cells (e.g., Phillips & Porter, 1977). These intracellular electrodes can record the synaptic potentials of single cells. The pipettes can be filled with materials, such as horseradish peroxidase, which spread into the finest dendrites and axons when injected into the cytoplasm of the single cell (Kitai et al., 1976). In this way, the detailed microanatomy of identified single cells whose receptive fields are known can be determined.

SINGLE-UNIT BRAIN STIMULATION?

The impossible challenge for scientists using electrical stimulation in the 1960s and 1970s was to match the rapid progress made in recording from the brain. The primary difficulty was that stimulation of single neurons in the brain (other than motoneurons) did not usually produce observable movements or even muscle potentials. By the 1970s, it was clear that electrical brain stimulation research could not match the single-neuron achievements of anatomy and recording.

Microstimulation

The aim of cortical microstimulation is to stimulate the fewest neurons possible in order to define the neural elements of each response. The first success of microstimulation was to measure the minimum currents required to activate single cells (Wall et al., 1956; Asanuma, 1981). Single neurons were found to be activated by currents as low as 0.2 μA in ideal conditions. The most sensitive sites on cortical and spinal cord neurons were found to be the initial segment and the nodes of Ranvier of the axon (Gustafsson & Jankowska, 1976;

Motor cortex

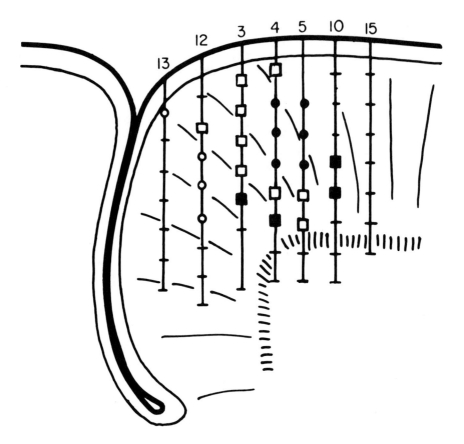

Figure 1-8. Microstimulation map of cebus monkey motor cortex (Asanuma & Rosen, 1972). Above, sites where movements were evoked at 5 μA. Open circles, thumb flexion; open squares, thumb extension; filled circles, thumb adduction; filled squares, thumb abduction; horizontal bars, no response.

Roberts & Smith, 1973; Stoney et al., 1968). The relationship between the current required for initiation of an action potential and the distance from the electrode to the site of activation was determined with great accuracy (Chapter 3). Furthermore, the spatial resolution of cortical maps improved by almost an order of magnitude (Figure 1-8).

Stimulation of the motor cortex at these lowest effective currents, however, failed to elicit motor twitches even at the highest frequencies of stimulation (Phillips & Porter, 1977; Asanuma & Rosen, 1972). To observe even the slightest muscle potential, currents of 5–10 μA were required in the most sensitive cortical sites mediating thumb, finger, or wrist movements. When stimulation occurred at the same time as a reflex, however, currents as low as 3 μA could minimally facilitate or inhibit a monosynaptic reflex. The size of the field of excitation or the number of neurons activated is still not precisely known in this case, but neither of these can be large.

If motor cortex units cannot produce behaviors, then which of these units, so carefully examined in recording studies, is important for motor behavior? This problem has tantalized electrophysiologists, who know that stimulation is the tool to show the links between units and behavior. In fact, Cheney and Fetz (1985) have recently gone to heroic lengths, averaging over thousands of stimulation trials, to show that the *probability* of a minimal muscle response can increase slightly at cortical currents as low as 0.5 μA, thereby increasing the likelihood that cortical units are involved in motor output.

PROBLEMS FOR BRAIN STIMULATION

Microstimulation of single neurons has helped to define the effects of current on cells and show that axons are the most easily activated substrates at the electrode. Microstimulation, however, has not resolved the basic aim of brain stimulation—that is, to determine which neural pathways and systems produce the behavioral response. For example, consider the most carefully studied case—motor cortex stimulation. Corticospinal axons in the pyramidal tract are an important pathway for the movements evoked by motor cortex stimulation. In primates, these axons make monosynaptic connections to spinal motoneurons serving the muscles of the hand and wrist, and these connections are clearly responsible for the fastest and most powerful movements of the hand and wrist (Phillips & Porter, 1977). Transections of the pyramidal tracts, however, do not block most stimulation-evoked movements, and sometimes even fail to raise the threshold substantially (Towe, 1973; Phillips & Porter, 1977). The extrapyramidal pathways that are most important in this residual response have not been determined (Phillips & Porter, 1977).

The frontal cortex sites that elicit eye movements in monkeys have also been mapped in exquisite detail (e.g., Robinson & Fuchs, 1969; Bruce et al., 1985). These "frontal eye fields" project to many other subcortical sites that also produce eye movements when stimulated (Leichnetz, 1981). It is still not known, however, which of these corticofugal pathways mediate the eye and head movements that result from stimulation of cortex. Consequently, 100 years after Ferrier's first maps, the essential pathways to motor neurons are not determined.

Furthermore, it is generally not clear which neurons near the electrode are excited by electrical stimulation. James Ranck (1975) made the point most painfully: "The phrase 'electrical stimulation of the lateral hypothalamus' is a shortened version of the statement that 'there was a stimulating electrode in the lateral hypothalamus which affected an unknown number and unknown kinds of cells at unknown locations in the vicinity of the electrode'." The excitability of neural tissue varies widely, so that estimates of the field of excitation found in one cell or one system cannot be easily extended to other cells or systems. Ranck argued that the understanding of electrical brain stimulation requires thorough understanding of the effects of stimulating single cells. He proposed a moral for all brain stimulators: "Think cellular."

There is little agreement about stimulation methods, also. Electrical stimulation can produce lesions or seizures (Isaacson, 1981), so there is much argument over which waveforms and electrode configurations are safest and produce the most stable results. The differences in methods make it difficult to compare the stimulus intensities used in different studies.

Neuroscientists want to know how brain cells and pathways put together actions, thoughts, and feelings. Usually, we must settle for understanding how simple reflexes work, often using simple animals. The "interesting" parts of the brain, however, are tangled webs of thousands of axons and cells connected by millions of synapses. Problems that are this difficult must be attacked by applying many converging methods, anatomy, electrical and recording stimulation, and chemical stimulation and recording, at many levels of analysis from single channels to whole brains.

AIMS OF THIS BOOK

The first general aim of the book is to review the fundamentals of neural excitation and apply these to brain tissue (Chapters 2 and 3). Along the way, suggestions for more standard methods of brain stimulation are offered. Principles of neural excitation should determine the choice of waveform and electrode configuration. Similarly, principles of measurement should constrain the choice of stimulation parameters. Chapter 2 discusses what stimuli to use and how to study stimulus–response relations. Chapter 3 considers the spatial effects of electrical stimulation.

The second general aim of the book is to describe the substrates that mediate electrically evoked responses (Chapters 4 through 8). The most powerful methods for describing populations of neurons are double-pulse methods that differentiate between the absolute refractory periods, conduction velocities, trajectories, and thresholds of different brain axons. In Chapter 4, the systems mediating self-stimulation and electrically evoked turning are described. For both responses, brain areas from the cerebral cortex to the metencephalon have been studied, and axon bundles responsible for the responses have been characterized. No attempt will be made to review all responses elicited by brain stimulation since only stimulation maps exist for most of these responses. In Chapters 5 through 8, the fundamentals of double-pulse stimulation are reviewed, with examples from single-unit and brain stimulation studies compared.

FURTHER READINGS

Ferrier, D. *The Functions of the Brain*. London: Smith Elder, 1886.
Human Neurobiology, Vol. 1(3). New York: Springer-Verlag, 1982. Special issue reviewing recent studies of human brain stimulation.

Penfield, W., & Jasper, H. *Epilepsy and the Functional Anatomy of the Human Brain.* Boston: Little, Brown, 1954. See in particular Chapter 3.

Phillips, C.G., & Porter, R. *Corticospinal Neurons.* London: Academic Press, 1977, Chapter 2. A history of motor cortex stimulation.

Valenstein, E., *Brain Control: A Critical Examination of Brain Stimulation and Psychosurgery.* New York: Wiley, 1973.

2

Stimulation and Measurement

If principles of neural excitation are to guide brain stimulation experiments, these principles must be discussed first. Neurons can be excited in many ways, such as by mechanically squeezing them, as we all know from the unpleasant experience of bumping our ulnar nerves at the elbow. Which stimuli produce the most reliable, countable effects on single neurons? What is the relationship between neural firings and the evoked responses? Although much of the material of this chapter reviews introductory neurophysiology or psychophysics, the goal of interpreting brain stimulation experiments remains foremost here.

EXCITATION OF BRAIN CELLS

Electrical brain stimulation requires a current source (stimulator), two electrical contacts (electrodes) for delivering and returning the current, and a living brain. Brain cells at rest have a more negative charge inside the cell than in the extracellular space. This negative charge results in a resting potential across the cell membrane of -40 to -90 mv. Electrical stimulation excites brain cells by reducing this resting potential (depolarizing the cell). A negative (cathodal) stimulus applied outside the cell or a positive (anodal) stimulus inside the cell produces this depolarization. The excitation of brain cells results in a rapid change in potential, first positive then negative, called an action potential.

Excitable channels

The excitability of brain tissue derives from special proteins, called *voltage-gated channels,* embedded within neural membranes. When the voltage difference across the membrane is reduced from the resting level, these proteins change their shape so that particular ions can flow more easily through the altered channels. The entry of positive ions, in turn, can depolarize the cell further, opening more voltage-gated channels.

In axons, the channels responsible for excitation are voltage-gated sodium channels. The simultaneous opening of many voltage-gated Na^+ channels results in an action potential. The action potential (which is also a depolarizing event) then opens thousands of Na^+ channels as it spreads the length of the axon. Although voltage-gated Na$^+$ channels appear to be the channels which initiate action potentials in axons, several other voltage-gated channels are found in axon terminals and cells, and so may also contribute excitation when these elements are depolarized. For example, the opening of voltage-gated calcium channels in axon terminals stimulates transmitter release.

Unmyelinated axons contain about 100 voltage-gated Na$^+$ channels per μm^2 of axon membrane. The channels are uniformly dense along the length of unmyelinated axons, but are especially dense (roughly 400 channels/μm^2) in the initial segment, where action potentials are initiated. Myelinated axons have their Na$^+$ channels concentrated in nodes of Ranvier at a density of roughly 2,000 to 12,000 channels/μm^2 with very few Na$^+$ channels between nodes. Na$^+$ channels are found on cell bodies at a density near 60 channels/μm^2 (Hille, 1981).

The number of channels that must open to initiate an action potential is greater than a few, since spontaneous channel openings occur without excitation. Each channel allows about 10 million sodium ions/second to flow through it when open, corresponding to 1.6 picoamps.

Current flow during excitation

The local stimulus that activates channels is a transmembrane voltage change from the resting level (usually -60 to -80 mv) to about -40 to -60 mv. The current flow is shown by the direction that positive charges move. Current must flow out of the cells through the resistance of the membrane and complete a circuit by flowing into the cell at a distance such that sufficient depolarization occurs near the channels (Figure 2-1; Ranck, 1981).

Anodal excitation

Extracellular anodal current can also stimulate axons. If the current flow is inward near the electrode, then outward current must flow at more distant sites along the cell. In myelinated axons, the outward current is concentrated at nodes of Ranvier, where the resistance is lower than between nodes, so that stimulation can occur at anodal currents ranging from one to eight times the cathodal threshold. Anodal excitation is sometimes called *next-node* stimulation, although the initial excitation may actually occur more than one node away from the electrode.

Oddly, anodal thresholds can be lower than cathodal thresholds—for example, when stimulating at or near the surface of motor cortex (Ranck, 1975). Surface anodal stimulation appears to produce inward currents at the top of radially oriented pyramidal cell bodies, and outward currents near the initial segments on the bottom of the cell. Since Na$^+$ channels are most concentrated near the initial segment, these outward currents can easily initiate action potentials.

A second type of anodal excitation, called *anode-break* excitation, can occur at the offset of a long-duration anodal pulse. In order for anode-break excitation

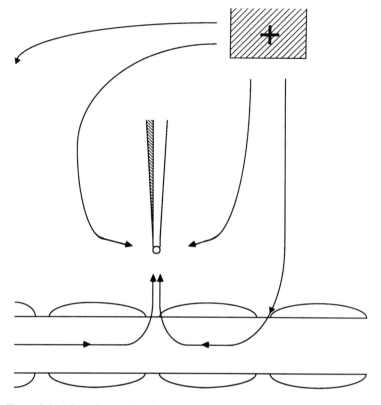

Figure 2-1. Schematic drawing of current flow during monopolar microstimulation of a myelinated axon. The stimulating electrode near the node is negative (cathodal) and the large return electrode at a distance from the axon is positive (anodal). Arrows show the direction in which positive ions flow. Outward current near nodes excites myelinated axons. Current flows into the axon at more distant nodes.

to occur, the pulse must be long enough in duration for accommodation to occur in the axons. The speed of accommodation varies widely in different axons, and the amount of anode-break excitation varies (Chapter 5). Anode-break excitation can be avoided by using a pulse offset that is gradual rather than sudden (Brindley & Craggs, 1980), or by using short-duration pulses.

STIMULI

The most efficient waveform for extracellular stimulation is normally a fast-rising, rectangular pulse of negative current (Figure 2-2). Cathodal stimulation is not only more effective, but is safer than anodal stimulation, which can damage tissue by emitting metal ions from the electrode. Furthermore, the excitation/lesion ratio is greatest for the fastest rise-time pulses. The maximum excitation can be compressed into the shortest duration if the time of offset is rapid also. Most stimulators deliver roughly rectangular pulses, so the current

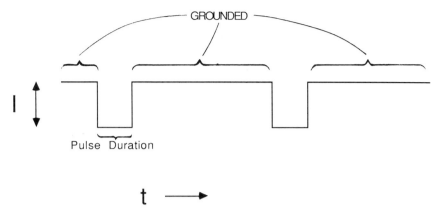

Figure 2-2. Monophasic stimulation is safer if the electrodes are grounded between the cathodal current pulses. The current return can occur through either the skull screws or grounded electrodes and is not shown here.

and duration can be most accurately measured when these pulses are exactly rectangular.

Short-duration pulses have several advantages over long-duration pulses. First, a pulse shorter than the absolute refractory period cannot stimulate an axon more than once. (Be warned, however, that short-duration pulses *can* excite several action potentials in pyramidal cells of the cortex, where many cells and synaptic loops are stimulated [Phillips & Porter, 1977].) Second, the time of excitation is better defined, since excitation can occur at any time during the pulse. Third, the least amount of charge is needed for excitation, which reduces the possibility of tissue injury. One-tenth msec pulses are used most often in paired-pulse stimulation studies, but 0.2 msec pulses are generally used in stimulation of the motor cortex. Stimuli longer than 0.4 msec should be avoided except for the special case where slow-reacting (i.e., "long-chronaxie") substrates must be excited.

Sine-wave stimulation has been used by many previous investigators. Sixty Hz sine-wave stimulation has disadvantages, however; the rise-time is very slow, the waveform duration is very long, and a long anodal phase (8.3 msec) follows each 8.3 msec cathodal phase. The number of action potentials per cycle cannot be estimated, the time of stimulation cannot be accurately determined, and the possibility of lesions is much greater than with short-duration pulses.

Stimulators

A constant-current stimulator, which delivers constant-current pulses, should be used rather than a constant-voltage stimulator. Although the neural membrane is excited by a transmembrane voltage change, at the stimulating electrodes it is the current, rather than the voltage, that determines the size of that transmembrane voltage change. Constant-voltage stimulators hold the voltage *(V)* between electrodes constant, so the current *(I)* varies with the resistance *(R),* according to Ohm's Law, $V = IR$. The resistance of the brain tissue can vary due to glial growth, edema, bleeding, infection, or even electrical stimulation. When a constant-current stimulator is used, the shape of the current pulses remains more constant, and the effectiveness of the pulses does not vary with the resistance of the tissue if the resistance is uniform in all directions around the electrode.

Polarization of electrodes

Tissue damage can also result from one-directional (monophasic) current. If the electrodes and tissue are charged during pulses and then disconnected from the stimulator to terminate the pulses, a negative charge can remain at the cathodal electrode to cause a lesion. The most secure way to prevent this polarization of the electrodes is by electronically connecting both electrodes to ground between stimulating pulses (Figure 2-2). In this way, any charge will be quickly removed. Most commercial stimulators are not designed to ground the electrodes between pulses, so an additional transistor that connects the electrodes to ground is usually required.

Another way to prevent polarization is to add anodal stimulation after each pulse, a method called *biphasic stimulation.* One biphasic stimulus is an identical anodal pulse following each cathodal pulse (Figure 2-3A; Lilly et al., 1955). Another biphasic stimulus is achieved by placing a capacitor in series in the circuit, called *capacitance-coupled* stimulation. This produces an anodal capacitor discharge after each pulse and alters the waveform of the cathodal pulse (Figure 2-3B). This capacitor method ensures that the anodal charge exactly balances the cathodal charge. These anodal stimuli seriously decrease the effectiveness of the cathodal pulse (Katz, 1939; Doty & Bartlett, 1981), and can stimulate the tissue themselves a second time (Chapter 5). Using biphasic pulses, then, the current of the cathodal pulses does not accurately measure the excitatory effectiveness of the pulses.

On the other hand, chemical changes can also occur at the electrode tip, and these are not removed by grounding the electrodes. The most damaging of these chemical changes are metal ions (especially iron) which are deposited at the anodal electrode. For this reason, it is safer to use electrode metals, such as platinum, which are not deposited into the tissue when current is passed. This reaction is reversed by biphasic stimulation. Also, hydrolysis of water produces hydrogen, which is very toxic, at the cathode, and oxygen, which is less toxic at the anode. Once hydrolysis has occurred, this reaction is not reversible by grounding or biphasic stimuli. Unfortunately, the rate of hydrogen removal in neural tissue is not known accurately, so the possible damaging effects are not well defined.

Therefore, two schools of thought still exist on stimulation. One school says that the possible chemical effects of cathodal stimulation should be reversed by immediately delivering equal and opposite anodal stimulation at the same site, and that grounding the electrodes fails to reverse the chemical effects. This

A

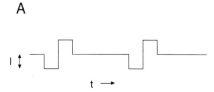

B

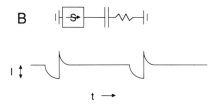

Figure 2-3. Biphasic stimuli. A. Each cathodal rectangular pulse is followed by an identical anodal pulse. B. Capacitance coupled-stimuli. The capacitor placed in series with the animal (resistor) returns all current when the voltage is removed.

school dominates the field of human cortical stimulation where safety is the primary concern (Girvin, 1978). The other school says that the anodal stimulation might also be dangerous and that the inhibitory effects of the anodal stimulation alter the effect and interpretability of the cathodal stimulation. This school dominates the field of animal brainstem stimulation where measurement is the primary concern. Although it is agreed that monophasic stimulation without grounding is unsafe and ineffective, it is still debated when monophasic stimulation with grounding between pulses is preferable to biphasic waveforms of various sorts.

Monitoring current

The presumed stimulation should be continuously monitored on an oscilloscope. An oscilloscope measures voltage, but current can be measured by the voltage change across a precision resistor (Figure 2-4). The current is the same anywhere in a series circuit, so the current can be calculated by $I = V/R$, where V is the voltage drop measured across the series resistor, and R is the size of the resistor.

Parameters of stimulation

Electrical stimulation usually consists of repeated waveforms, since repeated action potentials are needed to evoke most responses. To control these action

OSCILLOSCOPE

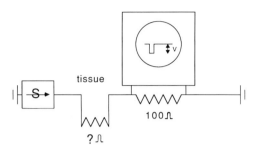

Figure 2-4. The current *(I)* through the animal can be monitored by the voltage *(V)* drop across a series resistor of known size, since the current is identical anywhere in the series circuit. In this case, $I = V/100$ Ohms, where *V* is measured on the oscilloscope.

potentials, the optimal stimulus is one that always results in one action potential per neuron recruited. Thus, the frequency of stimulation should be in a range for which all neurons can be expected to fire one action potential per pulse. For mammalian myelinated axons this frequency varies considerably, but in most cases is below 100 Hz for train durations up to 1 second, or below 20 Hz for longer train durations. For unmyelinated axons a lower frequency should be used. This one-for-one rule applies only for short-duration pulses applied to axons, since more than one firing can occur when using long-duration pulses, or biphasic pairs, or when stimulating the cortex.

Experimenters using microstimulation have often used only very high frequencies (200–2,000 Hz), so that minimal currents and small fields of excitation could be claimed. This is appropriate when high spatial resolution is the only aim of the work. At these frequencies, most myelinated axons fire near their maximum and are insensitive to increases in frequency. The number of firings cannot be estimated, so the frequency variable cannot be interpreted.

In most experiments, the variables to be manipulated are the current of the pulses, the frequency of the pulses (or its reciprocal, the interpulse interval), and the duration of the train of pulses. In addition, pulses are often presented in pairs. In that case, the first pulse in each pair is called the conditioning (C) pulse, the second in each pair is called the testing (T) pulse, and the interval between these two pulses is called the C-T interval. When trains of paired pulses are presented, the interval between pairs is called the C-C or interpair interval, so it is not confused with the C-T or intrapair interval (Figure 2-5).

Electrodes

Two electrodes are needed to pass current, so that a circuit is completed from the stimulator to the animal and back. If both these electrodes are placed into the brain, the stimulation is called *bipolar*. If only a single stimulating elec-

SINGLE PULSES

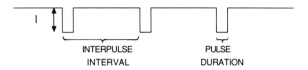

DOUBLE PULSES

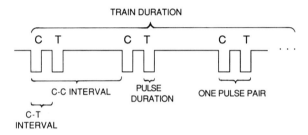

Figure 2-5. Temporal parameters of stimulation. Above, current, pulse duration and interpulse interval can be varied. Below, when double pulses are delivered, the first pulse is called the conditioning (C) pulse, the second pulse is called the test (T) pulse, and both C-T interval and C-C interval can be varied.

trode is placed into the brain and the current return is placed on the brain or body surface with a large screw or plate, the stimulation is called *monopolar*.

Bipolar stimulation has several disadvantages. If bipolar electrode tips are too close together, or if the insulation is imperfect, the electrodes can easily short so that no current is delivered to the tissue. When there is no short, it is still difficult to determine how much of the current was effectively delivered to the tissue. If, on the other hand, the bipolar tips are widely separated and the electrodes are fixed to one another or twisted together to allow accurate evaluation of the current passing through the tissue, a large scar will be produced by the electrodes as they are lowered through the brain. These problems are lessened if concentric electrodes are used in which the cathode is the central electrode and the anode is the surrounding electrode at a fixed distance, with larger surface area.

In addition, the field of stimulation is poorly understood using bipolar electrodes. During each pulse, one electrode is a cathode and the other electrode is an anode, so that cathodal and anodal stimulation of the tissue occurs simultaneously. When biphasic stimulation is used, anodal and cathodal stimulation occurs again during the second phase but via the opposite electrodes. The shape of the complex field of excitation is poorly understood in this case. Consequently, there is no way of estimating the current–distance relationship accurately with bipolar stimulation (Ranck, 1975).

With monopolar stimulation, the return electrode cannot stimulate brain tissue at normal currents because it is outside of dura and the surface area is very large. Since the return electrode is usually the anode, this monopolar arrangement also minimizes lesions and metal ion deposition in the brain near the stimulation site. The current density around the cathodal electrode dissipates uniformly away from the electrode (assuming a uniform resistance tissue), and so the field of stimulation can be approximated by spheres or ellipsoids of increasing radii (Ranck, 1975). Many current-distance estimates have been obtained using monopolar stimulation.

The only advantage of bipolar stimulation occurs when recording simultaneously. The presence of a return electrode near the source electrode reduces the current at longer distances from the stimulating electrodes, and thereby reduces the stimulus artifact observed at the recording electrode. In many cases, other methods of reducing the stimulus artifact are sufficient, such as stimulus isolation or disconnecting the recording electrode during the stimulating pulses to prevent saturation of the amplifying transistors. If these are effective, monopolar stimulation can still be used.

The practical design of electrodes and stimulators and methods for surgery and histology are discussed in Appendix II. There are many designs and methods that work effectively, so these issues are less fundamental.

Conclusions

The most effective stimulus is a rectangular, negative-going, current pulse less than 0.4 msec in duration. This stimulus minimizes the charge delivered for excitation, while reducing the lesion-producing effect of stimulation. Also, only one firing can occur per pulse in axons. The pulses should be delivered through a monopolar electrode, so that the size and shape of the field of stimulation can be estimated. Between pulses, the electrode should be shunted to ground to prevent polarization. Biphasic pulses that have a net charge of zero can be chemically safer than monophasic pulses and should be used when safety is more important than scaling of stimulus effectiveness. The frequency of stimulation should be moderate so that each pulse can be assumed to produce a single firing in the population of excited neurons.

PSYCHOPHYSICS OF BRAIN STIMULATION

Psychophysics is a branch of psychology that studies the effects of stimulus variables on sensation. Stimulus variables are chosen that best reveal the spatial and temporal properties of sensory receptors and integrative mechanisms.

Brain stimulation is a branch of neuroscience that studies the effects of stim-

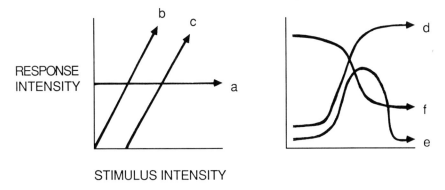

RESPONSE
INTENSITY

STIMULUS INTENSITY

Figure 2-6. Stimulus–response relationships. Linear (b) and scalar (c) relationships are rarely, if ever, seen. S- and U-shaped curves (d,e,f) are common, so that response intensity is not likely to reflect the amount of neural excitation accurately.

ulus variables on responses. Again, stimulation variables are chosen that best reveal the spatial and temporal properties of the biological transducers and integrative mechanisms that produce the observed responses. Consequently, quantitative analysis of the effects of brain stimulation parameters on behavior has been called the *psychophysics of brain stimulation*. Principles of psychophysical measurement can help in choosing appropriate stimulus and response conditions.

Stimulus–response relationship

Brain stimulation experiments begin by varying stimulation parameters and observing neural or behavioral responses. Neural responses can be unitary action potentials, postsynaptic potentials, evoked potentials, electroencephalograms, or electromyograms. Behavioral responses can be quantified by the strength or distance of movements or by the number of events recorded.

Once a response is defined, one stimulus variable is chosen and a quantitative experiment begins. A few types of stimulus–response relationships are shown in Figure 2-6. One common input–output relationship is that the stimulation has no effect (line a: $y = b$). A simple but impossible result is a scalar relationship; that is, all increases in stimulation produce the same increment in behavior (line b: $y = ax$). This is impossible because all behaviors require a minimum amount of stimulation to produce behavior; that is, they have a threshold. Also, behavior cannot increase infinitely, but has a limit in the amount that can be produced. This upper limit makes line c, the linear relationship $(y = ax + b)$ equally impossible. In some cases, a linear relationship is approximated over a limited range of stimulus intensities, however.

Most input–output relationships have forms such as lines d, e, and f. An S-shaped curve (d) is the result of thresholds and ceilings. High levels of stimulation can reverse the effect of stimulation, so that an inverted U-shaped curve results (e). The stimulation can inhibit a spontaneously occurring response, so that an inverted S-shaped curve results (f).

Order of stimulus presentation

The simplest method is to adjust the stimulation intensity near the level that produces the response of interest. This "method of adjustment" requires the fewest stimulations, since only the stimuli of maximum interest need to be presented and the order of presentations is not constrained. After the experiment, though, it is difficult to determine whether the results were affected by the order of presentations, so this method is dangerously susceptible to biases due to the subject or experimenter (depending on who controls the stimulus).

Stimuli can be presented sequentially from the lowest level to the highest (ascending order), or the highest to the lowest (descending order). This approach is called the *method of limits*. Previous stimuli can either improve sensitivity (warm-up effect), or decrease sensitivity (fatigue or adaptation effects). In behavioral experiments, the subject can anticipate the next stimulus when the order is predictable. Both the ascending and descending order of stimulus intensities should be used so that the size of order effects can be assessed.

To reduce order effects, the order of stimuli can be randomized or counterbalanced. Since this order cannot be changed once begun, the critical range of stimuli must be known beforehand. This method *(method of constant stimuli)* can be more time-consuming, since all levels of the stimuli must be delivered once chosen.

The method chosen depends on the accuracy required, the time available, and the estimated size of possible order and bias effects. No matter which method is chosen, the stimulus–response relationship should be tested often enough to obtain error estimates for all critical stimulus points.

Trade-off experiments

A more advanced experiment uses two stimulus variables rather than one. The effectiveness of one stimulus is measured, not by its effect on responding, but by its effect on a second stimulus variable. A sensitive response level is chosen (often, half the maximum response level), and the combination of two stimulation parameters required to produce this constant response level is observed (Figure 2-7). This is called a *trade-off experiment,* because the trade-off between two stimulus variables is measured. In trade-off experiments, the form of the stimulus–response relationship does not matter; all that is required is a monotonic relationship between stimulus intensity and response intensity in any range of stimulus intensities.

Trade-off experiments have several advantages over stimulus–response experiments. First, trade-off experiments are less subject to floor and ceiling effects. Both stimuli can often be varied over several orders of magnitude without serious variations in reliability. Since the response level is the same, the subject is not strained by extreme values of response output.

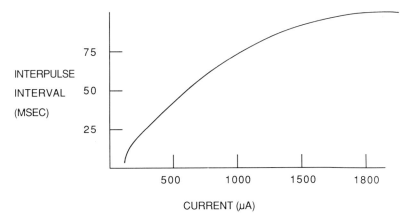

Figure 2-7. Trade-off relations. The curve represents the combination of two stimulus variables required to produce a constant response intensity. In this case, the combinations of interpulse interval and current required to produce three complete circles in a 10-second train of stimulation are shown (after Yeomans et al., 1984).

Second, because of the wide range of stimulus variables, the variables can be scaled or transformed in many interesting ways. One can make log transformations, reciprocal transformations, square root, squared, and so forth. The size of the range allows one to discriminate between these transformations and decide which transformations make the data clearest conceptually.

Third, trade-off relationships are relatively insensitive to performance variables, such as whether the subject is sick, how much training precedes the test, or whether the mechanical measurement apparatus is oiled. These variables can influence the reliability of the data or the absolute values obtained, but rarely influence the quantitative form of the trade-off relationship.

The trade-off relationship between two stimuli can be studied using many different responses. For example, in vision, the trade-off relationship between the intensity (number of photons) and the wavelength of light can be studied measuring rhodopsin bleaching, photon absorption, intrarod transmitter level, transmembrane potential, sodium current, electroretinogram, action potential rate, circadian activity, or "yes, I see it" verbal response. The stimulus–response relationship for each of these measures may be different, but the trade-off functions are remarkably similar. The similarity of these functions at low intensities suggests that these responses must have a transducer in common (i.e., rhodopsin) (Gallistel et al., 1981).

In brain stimulation, the parameters of stimulation can be similarly varied to establish trade-off relationships. For example, the trade-off between frequency and current can suggest the spatial properties of excitation in the behavior-producing neurons. The trade-off between interpulse interval and current for midbrain stimulation producing a circling response is shown in Figure 2-7. As the interpulse interval increases, the current required to produce a constant amount of circling increases. From this relationship, simple models of the excitation and integration of information in the neurons can be constructed (Chapter 3).

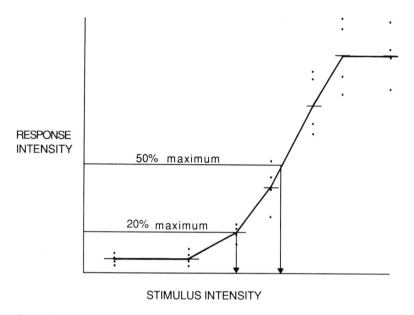

Figure 2-8. Stimulus–response curve. A stimulus presented several times evokes responses of different intensity. Since response errors are lower at lower stimulus values in this case, a response criterion just above minimum may be preferable to a half-maximum criterion.

Choice of response level

What fixed response level should be chosen in a trade-off experiment? In principle, the response level should be chosen that produces the smallest errors in estimating the stimulus intensity required to reach that criterion level (Figure 2-8). These errors are difficult to measure, however, since the observed errors are in response intensity, not stimulus intensity.

In practice, the half-maximum level is often chosen for the criterion level. If the stimulus–response curve is S-shaped, the best discrimination between stimuli should be obtained at that level. That is, the curve rises most sharply and the response error bars overlap least for equal stimulus steps at that level. In some cases, a lower response level is preferable because response errors are smaller near threshold than near maximum (Figure 2-8). In other cases, a low response level is preferred because the response stays reliable for longer periods, due to less fatigue, for example. It is useful to plot the entire stimulus–response function with error bars at least once to determine the best response range for discriminating stimuli.

Once the response level is chosen, the stimulus intensity required to achieve that level must be estimated by obtaining points above and below the criterion. Each estimate requires one point above and one below criterion. A line is usually drawn between these two points (linear interpolation), and the intersection of that line with the criterion response level defines the required stimulus intensity. Errors can be evaluated by making several such estimates. Stimulus in-

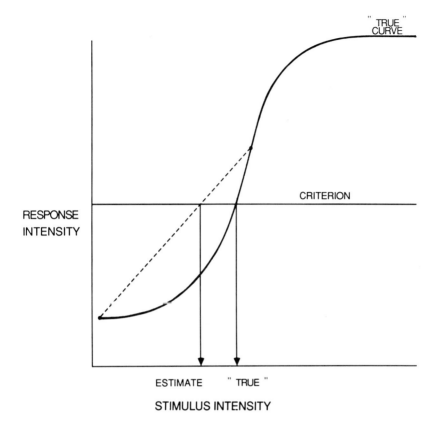

Figure 2-9. Estimation of required stimulus intensity by linear interpolation can be biased, since most curves are nonlinear.

tensities should be chosen far enough apart so that points above and below criterion are always obtained, but close enough together so that nonlinearities in the underlying stimulus–response curve do not result in errors due to linear interpolation. For example, if one point is in the middle of the S-shaped curve and the second point is at the floor, the estimate by linear interpolation will be lower than the "true" curve (Figure 2-9). In many cases, the stimulus variable is placed on a logarithmic scale before interpolations are made.

Choice of stimulus variables

Which stimulus variables are most useful for measuring stimulus effectiveness? Many variables are available to choose from: current, pulse duration, charge, train duration, frequency, and number of pulses. All of these variables increase excitation, either by increasing the number of neurons directly excited or by increasing the number of firings in those neurons.

Usually, increases in current or pulse duration increase the number of neurons directly excited by the electrode. It is difficult, however, to systematically vary the number of neurons excited for several reasons. It is not often known how the density of neurons varies with distance from the electrode. The directly excited neurons can either excite or inhibit the behavior observed. Even if the number of neurons could be measured, the different neurons could be weighted differently by their location; that is, spatial summation need not be uniform. Therefore, variables such as current and pulse duration, which alter the spatial size of the field of excitation, are best held constant so that the population of neurons excited can be held relatively constant.

The number of firings per axon can be measured more easily by varying frequency, train duration, or number of pulses. The effect of these firings on the response, however, depends on the temporal integration of firings by the postsynaptic networks of the system. Often, a long train of widely spaced pulses is less effective in producing a response than a short train of an equal number of closely spaced pulses. In this case, temporal integration is called *leaky* because the integration works like a leaky bucket—the bucket is filled less by pouring in cups of water spaced in time than by an equal number of closely spaced cups. A weighting function (such as an exponential) can sometimes be used to add leakage to integration.

To reduce the problem of imperfect temporal integration, the duration of trains of pulses should be fixed, so that the leakage (or facilitation) is the same in all conditions. The frequency of pulses at a fixed train duration measures the number of firings uncontaminated by integration over time, if the rate of leakage is independent of frequency.

Therefore, frequency is the stimulus variable of choice in most experiments. If the frequency is moderate so that all neurons fire once following each pulse, frequency variations alter the number of firings without altering the time of integration or the space of integration. Most of the trade-off experiments described in this book vary the frequency of stimulation to measure the stimulus efficacy of a second variable, such as a current or C-T interval.

Although frequency is the best variable available in most experiments, even frequency scales can be distorted. For example, if two systems are stimulated, both of which affect the response, and these have different frequency–response curves, the resulting curve can be a complicated function. The effects of frequency should be tested over a wide range of values (say 5 to 500 Hz) before assuming that frequency has simple or monotonic effects on behavior.

Also, the frequency scale is useful only when integration of many pulses occurs. For example, integration occurs only for a few milliseconds in the acoustic startle reflex (Yeomans et al., 1989). Since only a few pulses can be integrated in such a short time, the frequency scale provides very little information.

Conclusions

Response intensity can not provide a linear scale of stimulus effectiveness because of threshold and maximum response limitations in response intensity.

The relation between stimulus intensity and response intensity is usually S-shaped, or inverted S- or U-shaped. Therefore, trade-off experiments that vary two stimulus variables at a fixed response level scale the quantitative properties of the response-producing systems more effectively. In many cases, the most useful stimulus variable is the frequency of stimulation at a fixed current and pulse duration, since moderate frequencies produce a scalar increase in the number of firings in a fixed population of directly excited axons. The train duration should be held constant to prevent nonlinear temporal integration from altering the measure.

FURTHER READINGS

Katz, B. *Electrical Excitation of Nerve: A Review*. London: Oxford University Press, 1939. A classic on the properties of axons.

Ranck, J.B. Jr. Extracellular stimulation. In M.M. Patterson & R.P. Kesner (eds.), *Electrical Stimulation Research Methods*. New York: Academic Press, 1981. The principles of excitation of myelinated axons are presented for nonspecialists.

3

Spatial Effects of Electrical Stimulation

Most behavioral responses elicited by brain stimulation require many firings in many neurons. These masses of neurons and masses of firings must be coordinated in ways that still allow determination of the properties of the single neurons that are involved in the response. Brain stimulation, as described in this book, is a statistical science that uses stimulation parameters to relate masses of neural excitations at the stimulation site to distally measurable responses in a quantitative way.

This chapter deals with the spatial factors that determine how many neurons are excited. The importance of these spatial factors to brain mapping is con sidered later in this chapter. Later chapters deal with the temporal factors that determine the number and temporal distribution of firings produced.

The stimulus–response relationship depends on three spatial steps: (1) delivering the current from the electrodes through brain tissue to the electrically excitable neurons in that tissue; (2) achieving a local current density sufficient to excite those neurons; (3) exciting enough of the right neurons to evoke the responses of interest.

RESISTANCE OF BRAIN TISSUE

First, consider current flow in an ideal medium. When the resistance to current flow is uniform in all directions, the medium is said to be isotropic. In an isotropic medium, the field of current density around a point source electrode is spherical, with each concentric sphere representing an isodensity surface. The density of current passing through a surface of unit area (that is, the current flux) declines with the square of the distance from the source (Figure 3-1A). Since the surface area of a sphere is a $4\pi r^2$, the current flux is the current at the source I divided by $4\pi r^2$.

Brain tissue, however, is a complex medium for current flow. The resistance of the many component elements varies widely (Table 3.1). These elements are distributed in many different arrangements in different sites.

These specific resistances do not vary greatly with stimulation frequency (Geddes & Baker, 1967). This implies that tissue capacitance is small (membrane capacitance is roughly 1 μF/cm^2), and that resistance is similar to impedance. The specific resistance decreases as temperature rises.

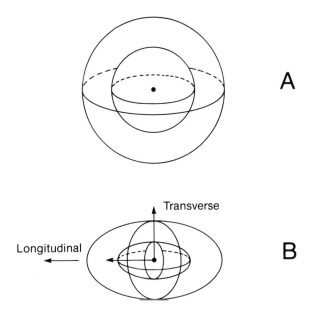

Figure 3-1. The current density field in an isotropic medium is spherical (A). In an axon bundle, however, the field will be longer in the axis of the bundle (B), due to lower resistance in that direction.

Current flows easily through cerebrospinal fluid, saline or blood plasma. Interstitial fluid probably is similar. The addition of membranes greatly increases resistance. In blood, the specific resistance increases from 50 to 300 Ohm-cm as the number of red blood cells increases, with an average value of 160 when the hematocrit is normal (40%). Cytoplasm also contains membranes, so resistance is similar. Gray matter has lower resistance than white matter due to the

Table 3–1 Specific Resistances in Various Tissues

Tissue	Specific Resistance (Ohm-cm)[a]
CSF, saline or blood plasma	50–60
Blood or cytoplasm	160 (range: 50–300)
Gray matter, average	300 (range: 200–850)
White matter, average	700 (range: 200–1,200)
Dorsal columns, longitudinal	200
Dorsal columns, transverse	1,200
Muscle, longitudinal	300
Muscle, transverse	1,600
Fat	2,800 (range: 1,000–5,000)

Sources: Geddes & Baker, 1967, and BeMent & Ranck, 1969a.

Specific resistance is defined as the resistance in ohms of a pure specimen of a given material 1 cm in length and 1 cm² in cross section.

[a] All measurements at 37°C and 1 kHz.

higher concentration of cytoplasm and the lower concentration of myelin. The highest specific resistance is in fat tissue, but the range is large, perhaps due to variations in the amount of fluid in and around fat. Fluid and membrane, then, appear to be the two primary resistive constituents of brain tissue.

Therefore, tissue is never completely isotropic. In the microstructure of brain tissue, current flow is easier along than across dendrites and blood vessels. In some gray matter, membranes are more or less randomly arrayed, so that the assumption of isotropy is a fair approximation when ventricles or large blood vessels are not nearby.

Isotropy is a poor assumption in muscles and axon bundles in which membranes are longitudinally arranged. The resistance is lower along than across the longitudinal axis. The ratio (transverse resistance/longitudinal resistance) varies from less than 2 to 9 in different axon bundles, however. The field of stimulation in axon bundles is better approximated by an ellipsoid whose major axis is in the direction of the bundle, rather than a sphere (Figure 3-1B). The ratio (major axis/minor axis) roughly equals the ratio (transverse resistance/longitudinal resistance). In the cross section of the bundle at the source, however, the current density field is still circular, as in the isotropic case.

The most important source of anisotropy in brain stimulation is often the electrode track itself. The electrode track is a puncture wound which often has a lower resistance than axons, so current can be expected to flow up the shaft more easily than into tissue. The puncture wound often contains fluid initially, but the fluid is then replaced by a glial sheath whose resistance may be close to gray matter. After several days, axons can regenerate around the wound (Foerster, 1982), which should increase resistance. Movement of the electrode or infection near the shaft can lower the resistance by increasing fluid near the tip.

SPATIAL PROPERTIES OF EXCITATION

The occurrence of excitation, as measured by an action potential, depends on the direction and amount of current flow, and therefore on the location and orientation of the electrodes.

Current–distance relationship

The size of the field of excitation is determined by the current–distance relationships of the cells near the stimulating electrode. The current–distance relationship is measured by moving a stimulating microelectrode in steps past a cell while simultaneously recording the activity of the cell. The current required for a single action potential is measured at many points along the microelectrode track.

In Figure 3-2, for example, the electrode was moved parallel to a myelinated axon in a bath (Tasaki, 1959). The lowest thresholds were obtained at regular

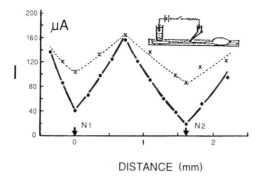

DISTANCE (mm)

Figure 3-2. Currents required for excitation of a myelinated axon by a microelectrode placed at different sites
along the length of the axon (after Tasaki, 1959). Current thresholds are lowest near nodes. Solid lines, cathodal current; dotted lines, anodal current.

intervals along the axon. These intervals corresponded to the locations of the
nodes of Ranvier, which were located 1.6 mm apart along the axon. The cathodal current threshold (solid line) was more sensitive to distance from the node
than the anodal current threshold (dotted line). This ratio between anodal and
cathodal thresholds was larger when stimulating near nodes of Ranvier and
smaller when stimulating between nodes.

When the microelectrode is moved near the cell body, the lowest thresholds
are obtained when stimulating in the vicinity of the initial segment of the axon
(Gustafsson & Jankowska, 1976). In ideal conditions of microstimulation, the
current thresholds near initial segments are near 0.1 μA, which is almost identical to the lowest thresholds near nodes (Roberts & Smith, 1973). The microelectrode must be very tiny, about the size of the node (<1 μm), and almost
touching the membrane to minimize the threshold. The thresholds for cells,
dendrites, and internodal axons are at least 10 times higher, suggesting that the
distance from the node or initial segment is critical (Gustafsson & Jankowska,
1976).

In Figure 3-3, for example, the threshold current for excitation was measured
as a microelectrode was moved perpendicular to motor cortex pyramidal cells
(Phillips & Porter, 1977). The threshold decreased as the electrode approached
the initial segment, then increased as the electrode moved farther away. For
each cell tested, the form of the current–distance relationship was very close
to a parabola $(I = K(d-d_o)^2)$, where I is the threshold current, d is the estimated
distance between electrode and initial segment, and d_o is the estimated minimum distance between electrode and initial segment (Gustafsson & Jankowska,
1976; Asanuma et al., 1976).

Current–distance relationships of many types of cells are shown in Figure 3-
4 plotted on log–log coordinates (after Ranck, 1975). The slope of the curves

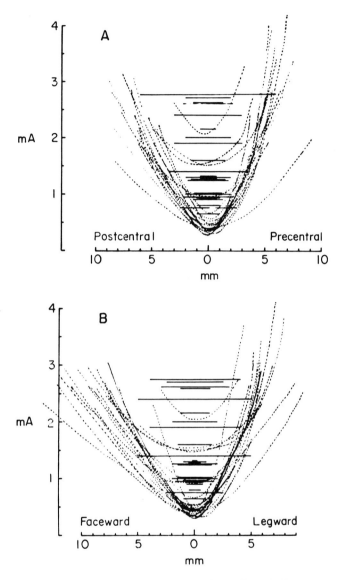

Figure 3-3. Currents required for excitation of pyramidal cells in motor cortex of baboon (Landgren et al., 1962). The microelectrode was moved parallel to the surface of the cortex, and so presumably perpendicular to the unseen cells. The lowest threshold point is taken to be 0 mm in all cases. Upper figure, anterior–posterior electrode movements; lower figure, medial–lateral. Each dotted curve shows the data for a single unit. Each horizontal line shows the width of the curve at the currents indicated for the cells.

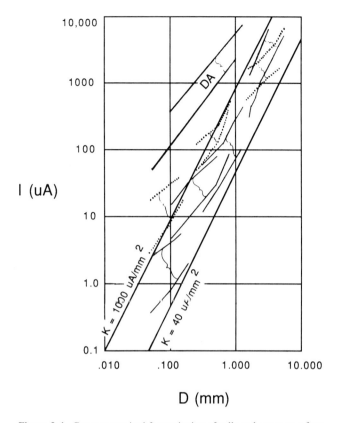

Figure 3-4. Currents required for excitation of cells and axons as a function of distance in studies reviewed by Ranck (1975). Both current and distance are plotted on logarithmic coordinates. For each study, labelled A–H after Ranck, a pair of curves is shown, with the lower right curve showing the lowest threshold neuron and the upper left curve showing the highest threshold neuron. The two long parallel lines (slope 2.0) show the predicted relationship if $I = Kr^2$, when $K = 40$ μA/mm^2 (farthest right line) and when $K = 1,000$ μA/mm^2 (line from apparent origin). Lines show minimum thresholds obtained, while shaded area show regions where higher thresholds were obtained. Current–distance data for unmyelinated axons of dopamine cells (labelled DA) are added (Yeomans et al., 1988). All data are based on 0.2-msec monophasic pulses.

indicates the exponent of the relationship. The long lines show the squared relationship, which closely fits the relationship for both axons and cells.

If

$$I = Kd^2$$

$$\log I = 2 \log d + C$$

and the slope is 2.

BeMent and Ranck (1969b), Bean (1974), and Hentall (1985) have argued that the current–distance relationship for axons should theoretically approach linear when the electrode is within 0.2 mm of a node, and approach cubic at very long distances. If this were true, the slope should approach 1 at very short distances and increase to 3 at longer distances in Figure 3-4. A few of the curves show a change in slope in this direction as distance increases, but others stay close to the squared relationship (slope 2) throughout. In any case, all data support the squared relationship as the best single approximation. In brain stimulation, where stimulation of many neurons at various distances occurs, the squared relationship is a useful rule of thumb but is not a strict law; however, only the squared current–distance relationship will be used in subsequent discussions of spatial effects in this book.

In the $I = Kd^2$ relation, the constant K, measured in $\mu A/mm^2$, describes the excitability of the nearest excitable membrane independent of the distance of the electrode from the membrane. K varies from 30 $\mu A/mm^2$ to 500 $\mu A/mm^2$ for large axons and up to 5,000 for small axons and cells. These estimates are based on 0.20 msec duration pulses, so to make estimates for 0.10 msec pulses, the K values should be multiplied by 1.7.

In an isotropic medium, the current flux *(F)* at any sphere

$$F = I/(4 \pi r^2)$$

Since

$$K = I/ r^2$$

the threshold current flux $F = K/(4 \pi)$. Therefore, K, the current–distance constant, is proportional to F, the current flux threshold, when impedance is isotropic.

Block

Finally, let me discuss two second-order effects of electrical stimulation: block and electrode orientation. Action potentials can be blocked in several ways. The easiest way is to initiate a second action potential. Two action potentials traveling toward one another cancel each other. This collision of action potentials will be discussed in Chapter 7.

Action potentials can also be blocked by strong inward current. This inward current must be two to five times the outward current required for excitation. Excitation usually requires only a $+ 10$ to $+ 40$ mv transmembrane stimulus while block of a full-sized action potential requires about a $- 50$ to $- 80$ mv hyperpolarizing stimulus.

This hyperpolarization block can even be produced by a cathode. The flow of outward current near a cathodal source results in inward current (hyperpolarizing current) at distance nodes (Figure 3-1). This hyperpolarization can occasionally block the conduction of action potentials (Ranck, 1975). Therefore,

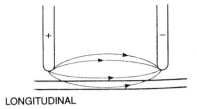

LONGITUDINAL

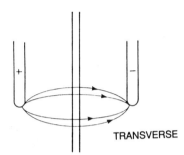

TRANSVERSE

Figure 3-5. Longitudinal stimulation is more effective than transverse stimulation (Ranck, 1981).

hyperpolarization block can be observed when cathodal currents above five times the current threshold for excitation are used. When stimulating a bundle of axons with a cathode, however, hyperpolarization block can only involve a small percentage of axons near the electrode at most. The high currents required to produce block always excite high-threshold or distant axons as well, so this effect is less important in behavioral experiments than in unit experiments.

Orientation of electrodes

The direction of current flow can also influence excitation. If stimulating current is delivered between two plates on opposite sides of an axon, the transverse current is the same along the length of the cell and so current cannot exit the axon easily. The stimulating current required for excitation, therefore, is much higher than normal. In the case of longitudinal current, the threshold current is very low, since current flows easily through the axon toward the cathode (Figure 3-5).

If bipolar electrode tips are placed along rather than across a bundle of axons, the threshold for stimulation can be slightly lower. The current is not as strictly transverse and longitudinal for all axons using point electrodes as using plates, however. Consequently, transverse stimulation has thresholds one to three times that of longitudinal stimulation using electrode tips, whereas using plates the current threshold for transverse stimulation can be more than 10 times that for longitudinal stimulation (Rushton, 1927).

Hyperpolarization block is also facilitated if an anode is placed near the axon. The anode concentrates the inward current and therefore blocks conduction near this anode. This block does not prevent conduction in the direction away from the anode.

CONCLUSIONS

Brain tissue varies in specific resistance, with fluid having low resistance and membranes having higher resistance. The flow of current depends on the arrangement of these elements. Gray matter can be roughly isotropic, so the current density field can be roughly approximated by concentric spheres. In axon bundles, the current density field can be roughly approximated by ellipsoids with circular cross sections. Blood vessels, ventricles, and electrode tracks, however, can alter these ideal forms.

The most excitable elements are nodes of Ranvier and initial segments. Therefore, axons in their various forms are the primary substrate for all brain stimulation. The current required for excitation depends mainly on the distance from these elements. The current–distance relationship is approximated by $I = K\ d^2$.

MAPS

The aim of most electrical studies has been to locate sites where responses can be elicited. Much of the appeal of brain stimulation derives from the creative display of stimulation sites. Woolsey's "animunculi" (Figure 1-3) immediately convey the gross layout and size distortion of the cortical somatotopic maps. But these drawings can distort and oversimplify the true local organization of responses, which often do not contain a single, continuous, two-dimensional layout of the body surface, as Woolsey (1958) carefully pointed out.

Spatial resolution of maps

The accuracy of these maps depends on several factors: the location of the electrodes relative to the behavior-eliciting and -inhibiting substrates; the size of the electrodes; the ability to differentiate between responses accurately and reproducibly; the type and level of anesthesia and/or restraint; and the choice of stimulation parameters.

The first maps of motor cortex were made with surface stimulation. The advantages of surface stimulation are that electrode tip position can be easily seen relative to surface landmarks such as sulci and blood vessels, and no physical damage to the brain results from electrode penetration. Large substrates with low thresholds, such as those mediating eye and hand movements in monkeys, are easily stimulated with surface electrodes.

The most sensitive sites, however, are in the deeper layers of the cortex. Smaller, less sensitive substrates are often masked or are harder to excite with surface stimulation. Consequently, the most complete and most accurate maps are made with depth electrodes, using low currents and small electrode tips.

Definition of responses

The quality of the map depends also on the choice of response. Movements can be operationally defined in many ways: for example, by whole limb displacement, generation of a force against a transducer, or electromyogram (EMG) recording. More current is required to initiate whole limb movements than minimal EMG responses. Even lower currents are needed to modify on-going movements, or to change the probability of an EMG response.

Competing responses or inhibitory systems often obscure the response of interest. For example, antagonistic muscles might also be activated resulting in less limb movement. Therefore, accurate spatial resolution of brain maps requires that minimal responses and minimal currents be used.

As another example, the response required for medial forebrain bundle (MFB) self-stimulation is pressing a bar to deliver brain stimulation. Currents of 100 μA or more are required for this response. Stimulation of adjacent axons in the internal capsule produces lateral head movements that pull the animal away from the bar. Stimulation of axons ventromedial to MFB produces an aversive response that also reduces the bar pressing. Consequently, the geometry of the bundle that produces self-stimulation is difficult to separate from the geometry of competing systems (Gratton & Wise, 1983).

Restraint or anesthesia can also alter responding. If stereotaxic restraint is used, head and neck movements are greatly inhibited. The position of the body relative to gravity can alter the visibility of responses. Although most cortical stimulation maps are now obtained from unanesthetised animals, some subcortical responses, such as locomotion elicited from brainstem stimulation, are easier to observe with light anesthesia (Sinnamon, 1984). As the old song goes, "A good map is hard to find".

The best maps of motor cortex show that the somatotopic map is not fixed, but varies in its detailed organization from animal to animal (Neafsey et al., 1986). In this respect the cortex appears to be among the most plastic brain areas, an idea disturbing to mappers but consistent with the higher functions of cortex.

How many neurons must be stimulated to elicit behavior?

In humans, activation of one neuron can sometimes evoke perceptible sensations under ideal conditions. For example, if a microelectrode is inserted directly into a human peripheral nerve, stimulation at currents of 0.6 to 5.0 μA can result in a localized touch sensation (Vallbo et al., 1984). The sensation has a discrete current threshold, much like the threshold of a single axon. The skin area where the touch is felt has approximately the same size and location as the receptive field of the single axon recorded with the same electrode. Therefore, the localized touch results from stimulation of one axon.

The eye is even more sensitive. When human subjects are adapted to the dark for over half an hour, stimulation of the retina with as few as seven photons results in localized visual sensations (Hecht et al., 1942). These sensations are believed to be due to single photons altering single rhodopsin molecules in seven receptors. Even in the total absence of light, visual sensations occasionally occur. The rate of these "spontaneous" sensations is believed to be related to the rate of spontaneous isomerizations of rhodopsin at body temperature (Baylor et al., 1980).

In motor systems, human subjects are able to control single alpha motor neurons when given appropriate feedback from electrodes in the muscle. In the monkey motor cortex, microstimulation currents of 3 μA can lower the threshold for limb movements (Asanuma & Rosen, 1972), but alone do not produce observable movements. Therefore, very few cortical neurons (certainly less than 10) are needed to alter movement thresholds, but more neurons must be stimulated to produce observable movements.

In the periphery, visible muscle twitches can be elicited by activation of single large axons. These large axons are the first to be activated by electrical stimulation. Large peripheral axons, however, are usually the last to be activated by normal brain activity, motor cortex stimulation, or reflexes. This is called *Henneman's size principle,* which states that small motor units are recruited first and large motor units are recruited last (Henneman et al., 1965; Hess et al., 1987). Therefore, the recruitment order in extracellular stimulation (large axons first, small last) is exactly the opposite of the recruitment order following natural peripheral stimulation or cortical stimulation (small units first, large units last).

Trade-off experiments

Most maps are made by moving electrodes through brain tissue. Often the stimulus intensity is held constant and all observed responses are reported. In other cases, the current is varied at each electrode position until a criterion response is obtained. If maximum spatial resolution is sought, minimum currents should be delivered through microelectrodes, and very high frequencies of stimulation used to evoke minimal responses.

Changes in response type or intensity, or in required current, are less interpretable quantitatively than changes in required frequency, however (Chapter 2). Therefore, if spatial resolution is not the only goal, a second method is to hold the criterion response at a reliable constant level and measure the frequency required to produce that response (e.g., Miliaressis et al., 1983). Other stimulus parameters should be set so that frequencies are in a range that the relevant axons can follow easily, usually 10–50 Hz. If more than one response is under study, the required frequency should be measured for each response at each electrode position, if possible.

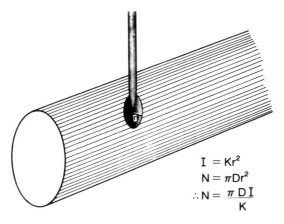

$$I = Kr^2$$
$$N = \pi D r^2$$
$$\therefore N = \frac{\pi D I}{K}$$

Figure 3-6. Model of field of excitation in a bundle of axons. The number of axons excited *(N)* is proportional to the current if $I = Kr^2$, and if K is the same for all axons.

THE NUMBER OF NEURONS EXCITED INCREASES WITH CURRENT

To produce behavioral responses, many brain neurons must be excited in most cases. How does the number of axons excited in a longitudinal bundle increase with current? This relation depends on many factors, such as the density and distribution of axons, the thresholds of the axons, and the electrode tip diameter. In the simple case of an ideal bundle of identical axons, the number of axons increases with current in a linear fashion, as argued shortly. The following exercises are optional, and impatient readers may wish to skip to the conclusions.

Model of ideal bundle

Assume that (1) all axons travel in the same direction; (2) all axons have the same threshold; (3) all axons are uniformly distributed around a point source electrode; and (4) the impedance transverse to the bundle is uniform. These assumptions provide a model of a "homogeneous bundle," a model that will be used several times in this book. Excitation occurs in all axons for which the current density exceeds threshold. The current density is constant along an ellipsoidal surface, as discussed earlier. The current density is highest for each axon in the circular cross section of the ellipsoid at the electrode (Figure 3-6). The field of excitation of a homogeneous bundle, then, is the intersection of the bundle and the circle with the threshold current density.

The area of the circle is expressed as

$$A = \pi r^2$$

Since

$$I = Kr^2$$

$$A = \pi\, I/K$$

The number of axons stimulated is proportional to the area of the circle. If the axons are distributed with density D (axons/mm^2), the number of axons stimulated is

$$N = DA$$

Therefore,

$$N = \pi\, D\, I/K$$

In this simple case, then, the number of axons stimulated by a single pulse increases directly with the current. In Figure 3-7, N and I are plotted as a line from the origin with slope $\pi\, (D/K)$. The slope increases as the density increases, and decreases as the threshold increases (Shizgal & Schindler, in preparation).

Tip size

If the electrode tip occupies a finite region in the center of the field, fewer axons are available in a given cross section to be stimulated, and so the threshold for stimulation rises. If the tip is a sphere of radius r_1, the area of the field is reduced by a constant, $\pi\, r_1^2$.

$$N = \pi\, D\, (r - r_1)^2$$

In this case, then, the relationship between current and number of axons is linear rather than scalar (Figure 3-7, dotted line; Shizgal & Schindler, in preparation).

The effect of tip size is more complicated if the tip shape is not spherical. The maximum current density at the tip surface is determined by the surface area of the tip: since the resistance of the electrode is much lower than the surrounding brain tissue, current will distribute itself throughout the surface of the electrode if the resistance of the surrounding medium is uniform. Consequently, the minimum current, I_0, is roughly determined by the surface area of the tip rather than the area removed from the circle. In the tissue, however, the current density will be more uniformly spherical (or ellipsoidal in the case of axons), so that the fields of excitation will better approximate circles in any cross section rather than the shape of the tip, except very near the tip.

The effective size of the tip includes the glial ''scar'' around the tip in which axons are not found. This region is more difficult to measure than the area of

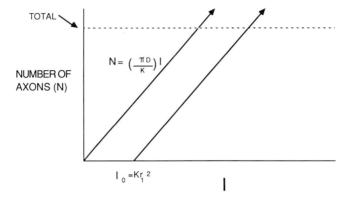

Figure 3-7. The predicted number of axons excited as a function of current. The current required to excite a given number of axons increases by a constant when the electrode tip diameter is increased.

the metal tip. In medial forebrain bundle self-stimulation, Milner and Laferriere (1986) found systematic increases in threshold with tip surface area. They also measured the glial layer around the tip to be 100-μm thick. Shizgal et al. (1979) found increases in thresholds following a small lesion made at the tip, but these increases were not maintained when tested over days, perhaps due to regeneration of MFB fibers (Foerster, 1982).

The number of axons removed by the insulated shaft of the electrode is not as large as shown by a drawing of the perpendicular shaft in a cross section. Although the shaft of the electrode must deflect axons to pass around it, the shaft does not substantially increase the minimum distance of the axons from the tip. Similarly, the angle of the shaft through the tissue should not alter threshold substantially, unless the shaft creates a low resistance path for current flow. The size of the shaft and the bending of the axons around the tip, therefore, have not been considered in this model.

Cylindrical bundle of axons

Axon bundles are usually limited to a small field. If the electrode tip is in the center of a field of axons of radius r_2, no further axons will be stimulated when the current exceeds Kr_2^2 (dashed line, Figure 3-7).

Location of electrode in field

When the electrode is not placed exactly in the center of the bundle, the number of axons stimulated depends on the area of intersection of two circles: the circle of axons in cross section, and the circle around the electrode defined by $I = Kr^2$ (Figure 3-8, left). For electrodes inside the field of axons, the number of axons stimulated rises linearly with current until the closest edge of the bundle is reached. At higher currents, the slope of the curve relating the num-

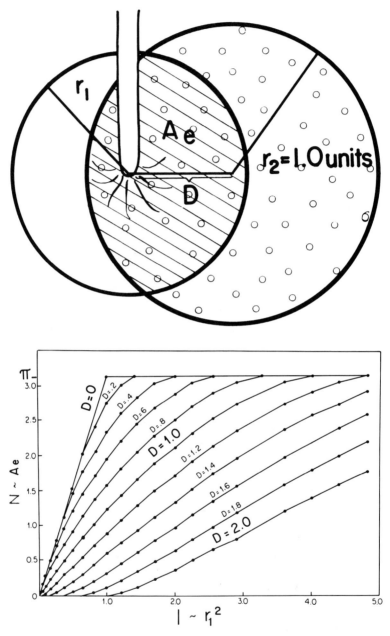

Figure 3-8. If the electrode tip is located off the center of the bundle, the relation between current and number of axons is nonlinear according to the model (Yeomans et al., 1984). *D* is the distance from the center of the bundle to the electrode, measured in units of the radius of the bundle (r_2). A_e is the area of intersection between the bundle and the field of stimulation.

ber of axons to current decreases. For electrodes outside of the field, a finite current is required before axons on the radius are stimulated. At higher currents, increases in current increase the number of axons stimulated very slowly. On Figure 3-8, $D = 0$ represents an electrode in the center of the field of axons, $D = 0.5$ represents an electrode halfway between center and radius, $D = 1.0$ represents an electrode exactly on the edge, and $D = 1.5$ represents an electrode one-half radius outside of the bundle.

Trade-off between current and frequency

Does this ideal model work for real brain stimulation data? First, an assumption about the spatial summation of action potentials over time and space is required to make a prediction for behavioral results. The simplest assumption is the "counter model," according to which the response intensity (R) is determined by the total number of firings (N firings), where N firings $= (N$ axons$) (N$ firings/axon). When response strength is held constant, as in a trade-off experiment, N firings is constant and, thus,

$$N \text{ axons} \sim 1/N \text{ firings per axon}$$

At moderate frequencies,

$$N \text{ firings/axon} = \text{pulse frequency} = 1/\text{interpulse interval}$$

Therefore,

$$N \text{ axons} \sim \text{interpulse interval}$$

Consequently, the spatial model can be tested by the trade-off between current and interpulse interval when the counter model is approximated (Yeomans et al., 1984).

The trade-off between current and interpulse interval for circling elicited by midbrain stimulation is shown in Figure 3-9. Each curve represents data from a single electrode. Electrodes placed near the estimated center of this bundle produced curves that rose quickly and nearly linearly before approaching asymptote. Electrodes placed a distance from the estimated center produced curves that rose much more slowly. These data were fit to the theoretical curves of Figure 3-8. From this fit it was estimated that 750 μA activated the entire bundle when electrodes were placed centrally.

At interpulse intervals below 5 msec, the data did not fit the geometric model. This effect occured independent of the current threshold for each electrode (Figure 3-9, bottom). At these high frequencies (200 Hz) the added pulses were unable to affect behavior, perhaps due to failure of the axons and/or synapses to follow the high frequency.

At higher interpulse intervals, however, the data fit much better. The best placed electrodes fit the theoretical curve $D = 0.4$, while off-center electrodes

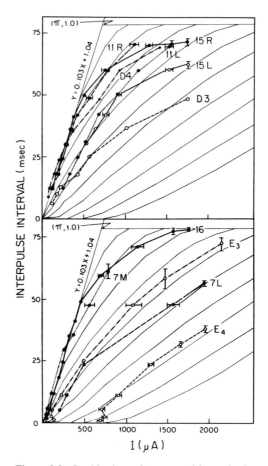

Figure 3-9. Combinations of current and interpulse interval required to produce a constant rate of circling in midbrain sites. Each curve represents a single electrode. These data are compared to the predictions of the model of Figure 3-8 (Yeomans et al., 1984).

fit theoretical curves $D = 0.7$ to 1.5. From the histological locations of the electrodes, the center of the bundle was located and the radius of the bundle was estimated to be 0.77 mm. Since 750 μA activates 0.77 mm, the average K of axons was estimated to be:

$$K = I/r^2$$

$$K = 750\mu A/(0.77mm)^2$$

$$K = 1{,}265 \ \mu A/mm^2$$

Therefore, the location of the center and the radius of the circling-producing substrate, and the current-distance relationship were estimated from this model. By fitting trade-off data to the theoretical curves, the distance of an electrode from the center of the bundle in radii can be roughly estimated in vivo in this brain region.

The one crucial variable that cannot be estimated in these data is the absolute number of axons. All estimates measure the relative behavioral weight of axons in different sites, giving relative estimates of density. To make an absolute estimate, the behavioral effect of stimulating single axons must be determined.

The conclusion of this exercise is that trade-off experiments can generate quantitative data that facilitate one's thinking about the neural substrates for stimulation-evoked responses. Current is a spatial variable that alters the radius of the field of excitation. The effects of current on the response depend on the location of the electrode tip in the bundle, the size of the bundle, the thresholds of the axons, and the radius of the electrode tip. Frequency is a temporal variable that alters the number of action potentials.

Limitations of model

The simplifying assumptions of this spatial model limit its generality. The cross section of the bundle could be more oval than circular. In this case, the current–interpulse interval trade-off is linear until the nearest edge is reached, but then curves more gradually toward asymptote, even when the electrode is placed in the center of the bundle.

Also, the axons may not be uniformly distributed inside the region. Inhibitory or conflicting effects from stimulating substrates inside or outside of the bundle may occur.

The current versus interpulse interval curve also bends gradually to asymptote, if the thresholds of the axons vary (Figure 3-10). In Chapter 7, evidence that the thresholds vary greatly is presented, so this limitation is important.

Because of variable thresholds and noncircular geometry, perfect linear functions such as $D = 0$ are not likely to be obtained even for electrodes perfectly placed in the center of a substrate. The current–interpulse interval trade-off functions can be influenced by too many variables to distinguish clearly between the possible alternative geometric models.

The current–interpulse interval trade-off can then, in some cases, estimate the placement of electrodes relative to the center of the substrate. Although this model can usefully describe the overall location of a substrate, a better way to map the local structure of a substrate is to use a movable electrode. Ideally, a low, fixed current is chosen and the interpulse interval is measured (Miliaressis & Gratton, 1981). According to the counter model, the interpulse interval measures the relative number of neurons activated at each location.

CONCLUSIONS

Accuracy of stimulation maps depends on many spatial factors, such as current, electrode tip size, location of stimulating electrode relative to the substrate, effects of neighboring inhibitory systems, and the sensitivity of response measures. These spatial variables have been optimized in microstimulation studies

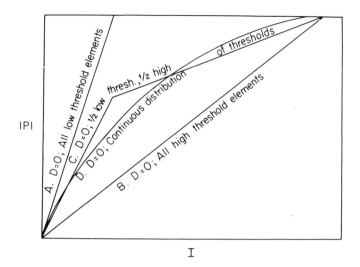

Figure 3-10. The predicted number of axons excited if the thresholds vary.
A. All low-threshold axons. B. All high-threshold axons. C. Half low-threshold
and half high-threshold axons. D. Continuous distribution of thresholds between low and high.

using tips under 5-μm diameter, with currents of 0.1 to 2 μA. Although humans can sense the activity of one neuron in ideal circumstances, observable
behaviors in motor systems usually require the activation of at least several
brain neurons at high frequencies. Another way to map brain regions is to
measure frequency thresholds for each response in a variety of sites along a
movable electrode track.

In a homogeneous bundle of axons with identical thresholds, the number of
axons recruited increases with current in a scalar fashion. Tip size increases the
minimum current by a constant for spherical tips. If the electrode is located off
the center of a cylindrical bundle, fewer axons are stimulated at high currents.
The number of axons stimulated can be predicted by the intersection of two
circles: one circle centered on the electrode with radius proportional to the
square root of current, and the second circle representing the cross section of
the bundle. The effects of these spatial variables can be observed empirically
by the trade-off between current and interpulse interval.

FURTHER READINGS

Geddes, L.A., & Baker, L.E. The specific impedance of biological material—a compendium of data for the biomedical engineer and physiologist. *Medical and Biological Engineering*, 1967, 5, 271–293.

Phillips, C.G., & Porter, R. *Corticospinal Neurones*. London: Academic Press, 1977.
Chapter 5. Reviews microstimulation studies of motor cortex.

Ranck, J.B. Jr. Which elements are excited in electrical stimulation of mammalian
central nervous system: a review. *Brain Research*, 1975, 98, 417–440.

4

Pathways Mediating Reward
and Circling

If axons are the primary substrates for electrical stimulation, then traditional methods of axon physiology—refractory period tests, collision tests, strength-duration tests—can be used to study the brain axons mediating stimulation-elicited behaviors. These excitability tests show whether slow or fast, short or long axons are responsible for stimulation-elicited responses in any site. This simple idea has been the foundation of the new approaches to brain stimulation. The methods that have proved most useful are reviewed in Chapters 5 to 8.

Before delving into that technical material, it would help to see how these stimulation methods have benefitted the study of the brain. In this chapter, an overview of two brain systems—self-stimulation and stimulation-elicited circling—is presented. First, the behaviors evoked by stimulation are described. Then, the effects of double-pulse stimulation are related to the anatomical and physiological properties of neurons in these sites.

BRAIN STIMULATION REWARD

A "reward" is any stimulus, such as a drug, food, or a mirror, that an animal will work to obtain. Rewarding stimuli are of interest because of their central importance to positive affect ("pleasure"), learning, and drug abuse (Stellar & Stellar, 1986).

Olds and Milner (1954) showed that rats will work to obtain electrical stimulation of deep brain sites, either by pressing a lever (Figure 4-1), or by returning to a location associated with the stimulation. Animals will also work to obtain opiate and stimulant drugs, such as heroin and cocaine, in several of the same deep brain sites. This suggests that brain stimulation reward may be related to drug reward (Olds & Fobes, 1981).

Intracranial self-stimulation has been studied in dozens of species from goldfish to humans. The similar sites where brain stimulation reward has been observed suggest that the structural organization of reward in the brain can be studied by mapping brain sites where self-stimulation is observed.

Self-stimulation can be obtained in electrode sites comprising about one fifth

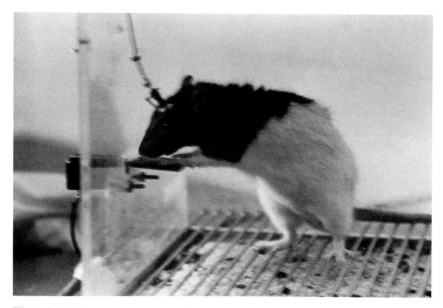

Figure 4-1. Self-stimulation in the rat. Every time the rat depresses the lever in the front of the box, a stimulator delivers a short train of electrical stimulation to the rat's brain via the wires into the box.

of rat brain volume, including sites as rostral as the frontal cortex and olfactory bulb to sites as caudal as the medulla and cerebellum. Stimulation of the medial forebrain bundle (MFB) evokes sniffing, exploration, and increased activity, all of which are signs of positive affect. In some sites, such as the MFB, acquisition of the response occurs in a few minutes, and the self-stimulation is vigorous, with bar-pressing rates commonly above 60/minute. In most brain sites, however, acquisition of bar-pressing takes several hours, and bar-pressing rates are nearer 10/minute. In each brain area, a characteristic pattern of acquisition, sniffing, locomotion, and posture is observed (e.g., Yeomans, 1982). Oddly enough, self-stimulation never satiates; that is, animals will bar-press for hours on end without slowing down in the least (Olds & Milner, 1954).

In spite of the variety of behaviors observed, early theorists tried to link all of these sites by one anatomical or neurochemical system. One idea was that self-stimulation is due to stimulation of the "MFB and all its direct connections" (Gallistel, 1973). The MFB has connections with dozens of different structures in all divisions of the brain, most of which support self-stimulation (Niewenhuys et al., 1982) (Figure 4-2). These connections, however, are too complex to allow cellular analysis of all connections.

The hypothesis that self-stimulation is due only to the activation of catecholamine-containing axons passing through MFB (Figure 4-3) was more exciting (Stein, 1975). The catecholamine hypothesis provided a specific anatomical hypothesis that could be tested by both traditional mapping and lesion methods and by pharmacological challenges. Norepinephrine- and dopamine-

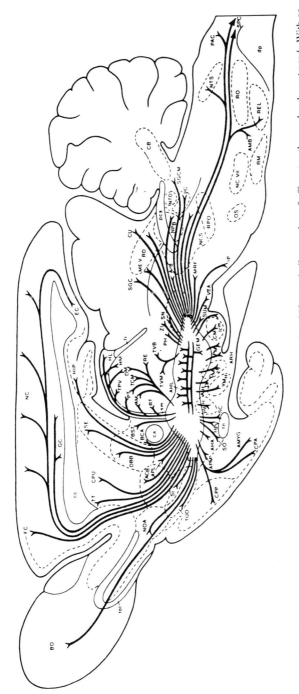

Figure 4-2. Efferent pathways of the medial forebrain bundle (Niewenhuys et al., 1982). A similar number of afferent pathways has been traced. With so many pathways, it is difficult to determine which pathway is critical for electrically evoked responses from the MFB.

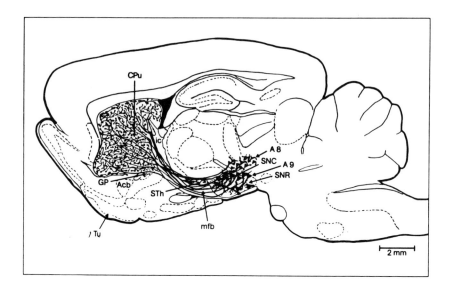

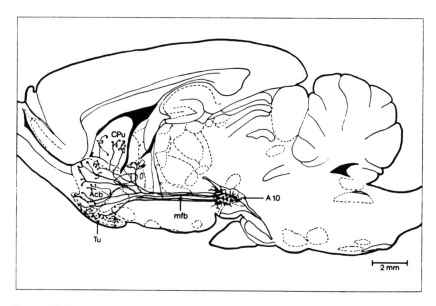

Figure 4-3. Dopaminergic pathways of the rat MFB (Fuxe et al., 1985). Upper, nigrostriatal pathway; lower, mesolimbic pathway.

containing cells were recorded from and found to have characteristic electro-physiological and pharmacological properties, which allowed them to be differentiated from neighboring cells (Bunney et al., 1973; Grace & Bunney, 1983; Chu & Bloom, 1973).

Dopamine-containing axons of the mesolimbic and nigrostriatal pathways have proved to be especially good candidates (Phillips & Fibiger, 1978; Wise, 1978).

Drugs that specifically block dopamine systems (such as antipsychotic drugs) have powerful inhibitory effects on self-stimulation in most sites. The drugs that are self-administered, such as cocaine and amphetamine, appear to facilitate the actions of dopamine cells (Wise, 1981).

The dopamine hypothesis, however, fails on at least two accounts. First, many self-stimulation sites, such as those in the medulla, cerebellum, dorsal pons, and caudal midbrain, are not near dopamine axons. Furthermore, self-stimulation behavior is very different in different brain areas, and this is not explained by the hypothesis that only two dopamine bundles are involved. Because of the range of behavioral effects, there must be not just one but several reward systems that are somehow interlinked. Double-pulse studies have described some of these other systems, and their relation to dopamine axon excitation.

Refractory periods

Deutsch (1964) was the first to report double-pulse brain stimulation. He found that bar-pressing rates for MFB stimulation increased as the C-T interval increased from 0.8 to 1.0 msec. He argued that 1.0 msec is the refractory period of the directly excited MFB axons mediating self-stimulation.

The basic approach of the refractory period experiment is shown in Figure 4-4. Two pulses are delivered in a bundle of axons. The first pulse (C) evokes an action potential in a population of axons around the electrode. The second pulse (T) evokes an action potential only if the C-T interval is longer than the refractory periods of the axons. Consequently, the number of action potentials doubles suddenly when the C-T interval increases from just below to just above the refractory periods. This sudden increase in the number of action potentials at C-T intervals in the refractory period range can be measured by a sharp decrease in the frequency required to produce a constant behavior, when trains of paired pulses are delivered (Chapter 6). If the axons mediating the behavior have a range of refractory periods, then this range can be measured by the range of C-T intervals over which decreases in required frequency are observed.

Subsequent studies of MFB self-stimulation have shown that the absolute refractory periods of MFB axons mediating self-stimulation range from 0.4 to at least 1.2 msec (Yeomans, 1979). Therefore, the directly stimulated axons mediating MFB self-stimulation must be mainly small, myelinated fibers. In other sites, or in other behaviors, shorter or longer refractory period ranges have been seen (Figure 4-5).

Transmitters for MFB self-stimulation

The MFB axons of midbrain dopamine cells have absolute refractory periods that range from 1.2 to 2.5 msec (Yeomans et al., 1988). Therefore, dopamine axons cannot account for the 0.4 to 1.2 msec absolute refractory periods found for MFB self-stimulation.

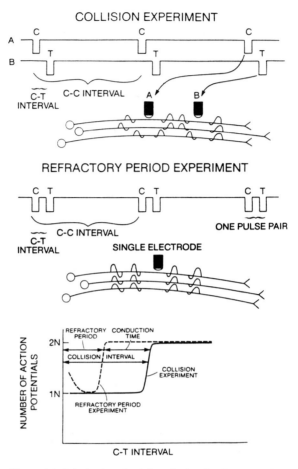

Figure 4-4. Paired-pulse stimulation of a bundle of axons. In both the refractory period and collision experiments, the number of action potentials in the bundle increases sharply as the interval between pulses (C-T interval) increases. The critical interval is longer in the collision experiment due to the conduction time between electrodes.

On the other hand, dopamine axons can account for the contributions of longer refractory period axons. The refractory period distribution for MFB self-stimulation widens considerably (0.4 to 2.5 msec) when small tip diameters, high currents, or long-duration pulses are used (Yeomans, 1979; Yeomans et al., 1985; Bielajew et al., 1986). This suggests that a second population of long refractory period axons (1.2 to 5.0 msec) is added when the current density is sufficient to stimulate high-threshold axons. The refractory period range of the added population is similar to the absolute and relative refractory periods of unmyelinated axons of midbrain dopamine cells. Furthermore, the high thresholds and long chronaxies of dopamine axons suggest that many MFB

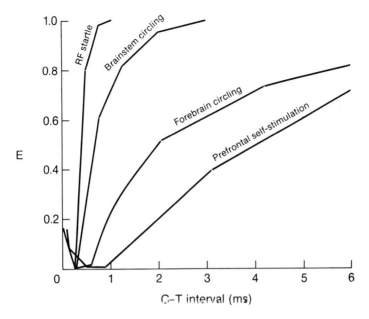

Figure 4-5. Paired-pulse stimulation of brain. The effectiveness *(E)* of the stimulation in reducing thresholds for the responses shown on each curve is plotted. *E* increased sharply at C-T intervals in the refractory period range. The critical range of C-T intervals varied for different responses and sites, suggesting that the refractory periods of the behavior-evoking axons are different.

dopamine axons should be activated when small tip diameters, high currents or long pulse durations are used (Fouriezos & Wise, 1984; Yeomans et al., 1988).

This idea has been tested by studying the refractory period distribution when dopamine blockers are injected peripherally. When large tip electrodes are used, very little change in the refractory period distribution (0.4 to 1.5 msec) occurs (Milner, 1975; Gratton & Wise, 1985). When small tip electrodes are used, however, dopamine blockers shift the refractory period distribution from a baseline range of 0.4 to 5 msec to a range of 0.4 to 2.0 msec (Figure 4-6). Therefore, the long-refractory period effects observed when current densities are high at the stimulating electrode are due largely to dopamine-sensitive substrates. These substrate are likely to be dopamine axons, but nondopamine axons may also contribute to the long refractory period effects.

The transmitter(s) for the short refractory period axons mediating MFB self-stimulation have not yet been determined. The most effective nondopamine blockers of MFB self-stimulation are anticholinergics (atropine, scopolamine, benztropine) injected into the region of the dopamine cell bodies (Yeomans et al., 1985, 1988). These anticholinergics selectively block the shortest refractory period axons (0.4 to 0.8 msec) either with peripheral injections (Gratton & Wise, 1985) or central injections. It is not yet clear whether these anticholinergics work directly by blocking short-refractory-period cholinergic axons in

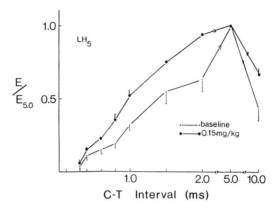

Figure 4-6. Injection of the dopamine receptor blocker, alpha-flupenthixol, decreased the contributions of long refractory axons to MFB self-stimulation (Krevs et al., 1987).

MFB or indirectly by blocking other neurons with muscarinic receptors in ventral tegmentum.

The collision experiment

In the collision experiment, C pulses are delivered via one electrode and T pulses are delivered via the second electrode (Figure 4-4). At both electrodes action potentials traveling toward the cell (antidromic) and away from the cell (orthodromic) are evoked. In the axons stimulated by both electrodes, the antidromic action potentials from the distal electrode collide with the orthodromic action potentials from the proximal electrode, thereby erasing half of the action potentials. The number of action potentials reaching the terminals doubles when the C-T interval is increased to longer than the "collision interval." The doubling occurs because the action potentials have time to pass the second stimulating electrode and avoid collision.

The collision interval is related to the sum of the refractory period and the conduction time between electrodes. The conduction velocity of the axons can be estimated by the interelectrode distance divided by the collision interval less the refractory period.

This collision result occurs only when the electrodes stimulate the same continuous axons in two places. Therefore, the collision experiment determines the axonal connections between brain sites, as well as the conduction velocities of the axons (Chapter 7).

Collision effects have been seen between electrode sites along the length of the MFB from the lateral preoptic area to at least the ventral tegmental area (Shizgal et al., 1980; Bielajew & Shizgal, 1982, 1986). Therefore, according to the collision model, self-stimulation is due to the direct excitation of long MFB axons which pass between the lateral preoptic area and the ventral tegmental area, with conduction velocities of 1 to 8 m/second. Bielajew and Shiz-

Brain Stimulation Reward

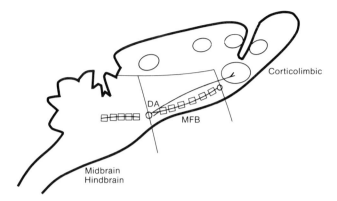

Figure 4-7. Sites where self-stimulation is obtained. Although many sites are known, only in MFB and midbrain are axonal linkages between sites known. Synaptic connections between these pathways and DA cells are still speculative.

gal (1986) have further shown that the direction of conduction is primarily from rostral to caudal. Collision has not been obtained, however, between MFB and other self-stimulation sites, such as the frontal cortex, ventral central gray, or dorsal tegmentum. Recently, collision was observed between the ventral tegmentum and dorsal raphe, providing evidence of a midbrain pathway for self-stimulation (Boye & Rompre, 1987; Shizgal & Murray, 1989).

Refractory periods have been tested in dozens of self-stimulation sites. In medial midbrain sites from the ventral tegmental area to the dorsal tegmental nucleus, refractory periods are very similar to MFB sites—that is, 0.4 to 1.2 msec (e.g., Bielajew et al., 1981; Rompre & Miliaressis, 1987). Summation between these caudal sites and MFB is also very high (Kofman & Yeomans, 1988, but collision has not been obtained in several attempts. In the lateral substantia nigra, however, refractory periods are much longer (1.0 to over 2.0 msec) than in MFB (Macmillan et al., 1985). These longer refractory periods may mean that dopamine axons are the main substrates in the lateral substantia nigra.

In cortical self-stimulation sites, refractory periods are longer than anywhere else yet measured (Figure 4-5). In the medial prefrontal cortex, refractory periods range form 1 to 8 msec (Schenk & Shizgal, 1982). These sites do not summate with MFB self-stimulation. Refractory periods in the dorsomedial thalamus and in the cingulate cortex range from 2 to 8 msec (Bielajew & Fouriezos, 1985; Silva et al., 1982). The substrates mediating self-stimulation in these sites must be much slower than those in MFB and do not appear to be linked either axonally or synaptically with MFB self-stimulation.

Figure 4-7, then, shows the present view of how reward sites are related. MFB self-stimulation is due to activation of a bundle that runs at least from the lateral preoptic area to the ventral tegmental area. The cells of origin have not been localized, although other evidence suggests the possible importance of cells in the lateral preoptic area, diagonal band of Broca, or lateral hypothalamus (Yeomans, 1982; Stellar & Stellar, 1986; Rompre & Shizgal, 1986; Velley, 1986). A second system of long-refractory period axons is activated at high current densities, and this system has the excitability properties of MFB axons of midbrain dopamine cells. A midbrain pathway for self-stimulation passes between the ventral tegmentum and dorsal raphe, and may or may not contain some MFB self-stimulation axons. Most midbrain sites summate well with MFB self-stimulation, and so may be linked by a synaptic connection. The proposal that this link is in the ventral tegmentum (at dopamine cells, for example), however, is not proven. Cortical sites are not linked with either MFB or midbrain sites.

RELATED STIMULATION-ELICITED BEHAVIORS

If MFB stimulation is maintained for many seconds, a variety of other interesting behaviors can often be elicited, such as feeding, drinking, copulation, forward locomotion, gnawing, nesting, hoarding, and killing (Valenstein et al., 1970; Hess, 1957). This rich range of behaviors has especially attracted psychologists and ethologists interested in the neural substrates of motivation, and complex species-specific behaviors. It is still not clear, however, whether these many behaviors are the result of activating separate neural pathways for each behavior, or of activating a single general motivational system that facilitates any easily available or "prepotent" response (Valenstein et al., 1970).

Soon after Deutsch's refractory period work, it was hoped that each of these behavioral systems could be distinguished by their refractory periods. Careful testing has shown that the refractory periods of several MFB-stimulation-evoked behaviors are similar to those for self-stimulation. The behaviors that have been tested are stimulation-evoked feeding, the facilitating ("priming") effects of MFB stimulation (Hawkins et al., 1983), and stimulation-evoked activity (Rompre & Miliaressis, 1980). For stimulation-induced feeding, collision also occurs between lateral hypothalamus and ventral tegmental area sites, with conduction velocities and trajectories indistinguishable from those for MFB self-stimulation (Gratton & Wise, 1988). Activation of the same fibers, then, may mediate all of these effects as argued by Valenstein et al., (1970), based on mapping data. Only for activity (Durivage & Miliaressis, 1983, 1987) and for the turning off of rewarding brain stimulation (Bielajew & Shizgal, 1980) is there evidence that different axons than those mediating self-stimulation mediate the behavior.

ELECTRICALLY EVOKED CIRCLING

The response most commonly evoked by continuous brain stimulation is lateral eye, head, and body movement, followed by circling. Fritsch and Hitzig (1870) reported that stimulation of a region of dog frontal cortex activated neck muscles. Ferrier (1876) found contralateral head and eye movements from a similar region in several species. Hess (1957) reported a variety of eye, head, and body

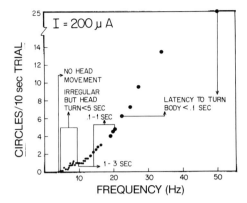

Figure 4-8. Circling evoked by stimulation of one midbrain site. The number of circles increased reliably with frequency. Each point represents a single trial (Yeomans et al., 1984).

movements due to stimulation of dozens of cat brain areas from the frontal cortex to the pons. In general, eye movements occur first, followed by head movements and circling. These lateral movements can be elicited in about one third of the rat or cat brain, including the parietal cortex, internal capsule, basal ganglia, superior colliculus, oculomotor areas, cerebellum, vestibular areas and pathways, and medial brainstem from midbrain to medulla (Hess, 1957; Pycock, 1980; Yeomans & Tehovnik, 1988). As in self-stimulation, the details of the behavior vary considerably from region to region.

The connecting pathways that evoke the responses were a subject of controversy for many decades. Several investigators argued that tectospinal axons are not necessary for eye, head, or circling responses from medial brainstem or cortical sites (Hinsey et al., 1930; Wagman, 1964; Schiller, 1977), but are necessary for contralateral eye, head, or body movements from superior colliculus sites. Many recent theories emphasized the importance of nigrostriatal dopamine axons in circling, but many other candidates exist (Pycock, 1980). No one was sure how eye, head, or circling responses evoked from cortical sites connect with brainstem pathways to motor neurons (e.g., Leichnetz, 1981).

Parametric studies of circling

The easiest sites to study with stimulation parameters are located near the midline in the midbrain and pontine tegmentum. In these medial brainstem sites, ipsiversive circling can be obtained at currents under 20 μA, for 0.1-msec pulses (Yeomans et al., 1984). If the stimulation is maintained, the circling continues at a more or less constant rate for many minutes. In this case, the rats look like they are "chasing their tails," but they don't stop unless the stimulation is turned off.

The rate of circling increases with the frequency (Figure 4-8), but can also be increased by the current as discussed in Chapter 3, unless inhibiting systems are activated. The stimulation parameters for the circling often remain stable within 10 percent over months of stimulation, if the electrode sites stay fixed, so there does not appear to be plasticity to this remarkable response. Consequently, this appears to be a simple and stable output system. Removal of the entire forebrain has no effect on the response evoked from the tegmentum (Hinsey et al., 1939).

Double-pulse studies of circling

When double pulses are delivered to the medial midbrain or pontine sites, recovery occurs at C-T intervals from 0.3 to 1.5 msec (Miliaressis, 1981; Yeomans & Linney, 1985). The initial rise occurs between 0.32 and 0.36 msec (Miliaressis, 1981), suggesting that axons with short refractory periods mediate this response.

Collision studies have shown that two pathways mediate the ipsiversive circling response in rats (Figure 4-9). The first descends from the rostromedial midbrain (around interstitial nucleus of Cajal) to the caudal pons near the midline (Tehovnik & Yeomans, 1986). The cells of origin and terminals of this pathway have not been determined. The conduction velocities fall in the 2-to-25-m/second range (Tehovnik & Yeomans, 1986; Yeomans & Linney, 1985; Miliaressis & Phillippe, 1983). In the ventral pons, the refractory periods and conduction velocities are slightly longer, suggesting that some slower axons are involved in these deep sites.

The second pathway begins in the intermediate layers of the superior colliculus, crosses the midline in the predorsal bundle, and descends in the trajectory of the tectospinal pathway through the midbrain and pons. The refractory periods and conduction velocities of this crossed pathway are similar to the uncrossed pathway (Tehovnik & Yeomans, 1986).

Circling elicited from the superior colliculus

The cells of the superior colliculus are separated into distinct layers. Visual inputs from retina terminate in superficial layers, making a retinotopic map on the surface of the colliculus. Inputs from auditory and somatosensory systems terminate in intermediate layers. These different sensory maps appear to be in spatial register with one another so that retinotopic maps align well with somatotopic and auditory localization maps. Maps of the direction of eye movements evoked by electrical stimulation show a similar spatial alignment (Stein, 1984).

The crossed tectospinal and tectobulbar pathway originates in large cells concentrated in intermediate gray layers of the superior colliculus (Redgrave et al., 1986). These cells send large myelinated axons across the midline in the predorsal bundle to terminate in many brainstem and cervical spinal cord regions (Grantyn & Grantyn, 1982; Rose & Abrahams, 1978). The conduction velocities of single crossed tectobulbar axons in rats range from 0.7 to 40 m/second (Yeomans & Linney, 1985). The conduction velocities suggest that the fiber diameters range from about 0.5 to 4 μm in diameter.

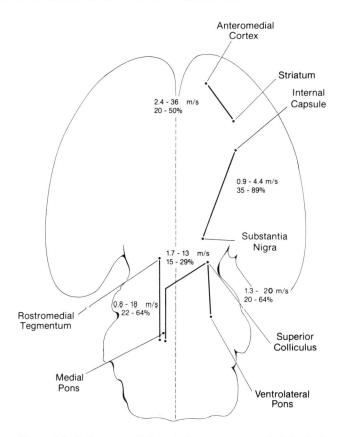

Figure 4-9. Pathways mediating circling responses evoked by brain stimulation. Collision is obtained along crossed tectopontine and uncrossed tegmentopontine pathways. Collision is also obtained along the striatonigral pathway, and between the cortex and rostral striatum, in sites where contraversive circling is obtained. An uncrossed tectobulbar pathway mediates ipsiversive turning. Collision is not obtained between any of the other combinations of sites. The conduction velocity range and percent collisions obtained are shown next to each bundle.

The lowest thresholds for circling are obtained with electrodes in the intermediate and deep layers of the superior colliculus. Even so, these thresholds are several times higher than in the contralateral midbrain and pons. This is partly due to the higher density of axons in sites where the two pathways converge into the midline midbrain and pons.

Cutting the predorsal bundle blocks the contraversive response evoked from the colliculus (Dean et al., 1986; Ellard & Goodale, 1986). Therefore, the collision observed between the colliculus and contralateral pons must be due to these crossed tectospinal and tectobulbar axons. The trajectories of the two converging pathways through the pons (crossed tectopontine and uncrossed tegmentopontine) appear to be similar using behavioral or anatomical methods (Tehovnik & Yeomans, 1986; Huerta & Harting, 1982).

Circling evoked from tectal sites is normally contraversive, but if the pre-dorsal bundle is cut at the midline, the head turns and circling are in the ips-iversive direction (Dean et al., 1986; Ellard & Goodale, 1986). An uncrossed tectal output mediates these ipsiversive turns. The contraversive responses nor-mally elicited from the superior colliculus are probably inhibited by the weaker ipsiversive response. The uncrossed tectal output takes a lateral path around the midbrain to the ventrolateral pons (Redgrave et al., 1987; Burne et al., 1981). Collision experiments show that the conduction velocities of the tectopontine axons mediating ipsiversive circling range from 1.3 to 20 m/second (Bucken-ham & Yeomans, in preparation.)

Circling elicited from the frontal cortex

The direction of circling when stimulating the cortex is usually contraversive, although ipsiversive circling has been reported in some sites (Sinnamon & Galer, 1984). In rats, contralateral movements are obtained from the most medial sur-face of the frontal cortex from the frontal pole to midcortex (Hall & Lindholm, 1974; Neafsey et al., 1986).

Circling is much less reliable in the frontal cortex than in the midbrain. As discussed in Chapter 3, the rate of circling slows down gradually throughout a 90-second train of pulses. The animals often stop circling and engage in some other activity, as if no longer affected by the stimulation. Very high currents (400 μA and up) are required for circling, and seizure activity often interrupts testing and alters thresholds over time (Tehovnik & Yeomans, 1987).

When a barrier is introduced into the path of movement, normal animals change their path to go around the barrier. During pontine stimulation, animals bump right into the barrier and slide past. If the rats are placed facing a corner, they are often unable to get out of the corner when the stimulation is turned on. Instead, they push steadily against the wall.

During frontal cortex stimulation, the rats back away from the barrier, often turning away from the preferred contraversive direction, before resuming their path. Rats, therefore, appear to be more responsive to external stimuli during frontal cortex stimulation (Tehovnik & Yeomans, 1987).

Double-pulse stimulation of the frontal cortex

Refractory periods obtained for circling in frontal cortex sites range from 0.6 to 4 msec, which is much longer than pontine or midbrain circling sites but still shorter than self-stimulation from the medial prefrontal cortex just 2-mm ventral (Tehovnik & Yeomans, 1987; Schenk & Shizgal, 1982).

Hess (1957) proposed that lateral turning in cats is due to a pathway between the frontal cortex and the diencephalon. He observed contralateral eye and head movements similar to those seen in the cortex in a series of sites immediately posterior to the genu of the corpus callosum of cats. Some of these sites are in the internal capsule.

In internal capsule and substantia nigra sites in rats, refractory periods are

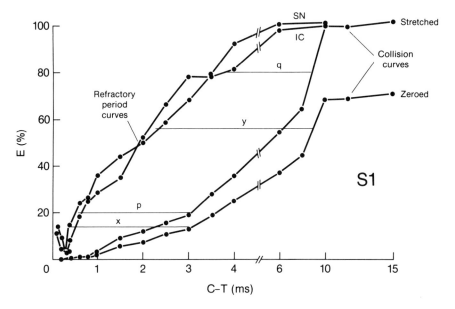

Figure 4-10. Refractory period and collision curves for stimulation-evoked circling along the stria-tonigral pathway (Tehovnik & Yeomans, 1988). Electrodes were in the internal capsule (IC) near the globus pallidus, and in the medial substantia nigra (SN). Currents were 100 and 400 μA, respectively. Note the long conduction times and refractory periods of this system.

very long (0.6 to 4 msec), as in the cortex. Currents required for a circling response are only 100 μA, or several times lower than in the cortex. Up to 90 percent collision is obtained between the internal capsule and the medial substantia nigra (Figure 4-10), suggesting that all axons in the internal capsule continue through the medial substantia nigra. The conduction velocities range from 0.7 to 4.0 m/second, which is very similar to striatonigral axons, but slightly faster than nigrostriatal dopamine axons (Richardson et al., 1977; Grace & Bunney, 1985). These conduction velocities, however, are much slower than brainstem axons mediating circling.

Collision has never been obtained, however, between the frontal cortex and either the internal capsule or the substantia nigra (Tehovnik & Yeomans, 1986, 1988). Furthermore, the trajectory and conduction velocities of these axons are consistent with striatonigral pathways and not with corticotegmental pathways. The output from the cortex to the brainstem is mainly through the rostral striatum, since collision is observed between the cortex and rostral striatum (Yeomans & Buckenham, 1988; Chapter 8). This suggests that a short cortical output pathway goes only as far as the striatum, and then relays via the striatonigral pathway to the midbrain.

The anatomical connections between striatonigral axons and the midbrain-pontine axons are not yet clear. Concurrent stimulation of any of the striatonigral sites and any of the midbrain-pons sites results in near-perfect summation, but no collision (Tehovnik & Yeomans, 1986). One likely connecting pathway is the nigrotectal pathway, which is a monosynaptic connection from GA-BAergic cells in the substantia nigra onto tectospinal cells controlling eye movements (Hikosaka & Wurtz, 1984a, b). These cells tonically inhibit the tectal output cells, so inhibition from GABAergic striatonigral cells (Grace & Bunney, 1985) could disinhibit tectal cells.

RELATIONSHIP BETWEEN CIRCLING AND LATERAL EYE AND HEAD MOVEMENTS

The sites producing circling responses are very similar to sites producing lateral eye and head movements in cats and monkeys (e.g., Bender, 1964; Hess, 1957) (Figure 4-11). In fact, when the body is restrained, the animal will turn further with its head and eyes. Similarly, when the head is restrained, the animal will compensate with its body and eyes (e.g., Guitton & Mandl, 1978). Hess argued that all of these responses are coordinated responses of orienting in space, not simply head, eye, or body twitches. The names "frontal eye fields" or "oculomotor systems," then, are too narrow and are misleading. Pure eye, head, or body movements are evoked only in the oculomotor and spinal cord nuclei and nerves themselves. Pathways for lateral eye and head movements in the brainstem, therefore, may be similar to those described here for lateral circling responses. Whether the same pathways will be found in different species remains to be determined.

CONCLUSIONS

Collision methods have defined the connections between sites where self-stimulation and circling are evoked. Self-stimulation of the medial forebrain bundle (MFB) is due to the direct activation of a longitudinal bundle of small myelinated axons, with absolute refractory periods that range from 0.4 to 1.2 msec, and with conduction velocities in the 1–8 m/second range. When high currents or small tip diameters are used, however, a second population of longer refractory period axons (1.2–2.5 msec) is added; the excitability properties of this second population are similar to those of the unmyelinated axons of midbrain dopamine cells.

Midbrain self-stimulation is the result of the activation of axons with similar refractory periods. Part of this midbrain self-stimulation results from a bundle of axons between ventral tegmentum and the region of dorsal raphe. Summation between midbrain and MFB sites is very strong. Frontal cortex self-stimulation is due to the stimulation of substrates which recover between 1 and 8 msec, but summation with MFB self-stimulation is poor.

At least five separate pathways mediate electrically evoked circling in rats, and different responses are observed in each bundle (Yeomans & Tehovnik, 1988). The refractory periods, conduction velocities, and trajectories of the axons mediating circling in each of these five bundles have been measured.

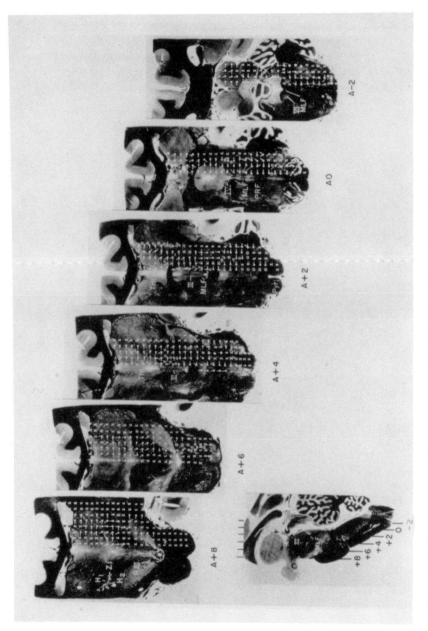

Figure 4-11. Eye movements evoked by brain stem stimulation in monkeys (Wagman, 1964). Data are shown on six coronal sections, from rostral (left) to caudal (right). The orientation of these sections is shown on the midsagittal section at the lower left.

FURTHER READINGS

Pycock, C.J. Turning behavior in animals. *Neuroscience*, 1980, *5*, 461–516.
Stellar, J., & Stellar, E. *Biology of Motivation and Reward*. New York: Springer-Verlag, 1986.
Yeomans, J.S. Mechanisms of brain-stimulation reward. *Progress in Psychobiology and Physiological Psychology*, 1988, *13*, 227–266.
Yeomans, J.S., & Tehovnik, E.J. Turning responses evoked by stimulation of visuo-motor pathways. *Brain Research Reviews*, 1988, *13*, 235–259.

Temporal Summation

Once a region is mapped, it is useful to determine which neurons within the region are responsible for the effect of interest. Since many neurons are excited in each brain site, location alone cannot determine which neural elements make the strongest impact on the observed response. Although axon bundles are the most likely substrates for brain stimulation, the directly excited elements that produce the response could be initial segments, large or small myelinated axons, or unmyelinated axons. Even cell bodies or local circuits could make some contribution. The temporal properties of these elements vary widely.

In the next chapters, the temporal parameters of stimulation are varied to help characterize the elements producing the response. In each chapter, the properties of single axons are first reviewed, followed by comparable brain stimulation experiments observing behavior. Axonal temporal characteristics are usually measured in tenths of milliseconds, since electricity moves rapidly through tissue, and voltage-gated channels recover quickly from excitation. Consequently, the microsecond timing of electrical stimuli can alter the number of firings produced in each of the directly excited elements. Synaptic integration is usually much slower.

In Chapter 3, the effects of fixed duration trains of equally spaced 0.1-msec pulses were considered. In this chapter, the summation times of systems are measured (1) by varying the duration of each pulse, (2) by presenting paired pulses or (3) by varying the duration of trains of pulses. Paired pulses will be used to study refractory periods in Chapter 6.

The methods discussed in this chapter are not generally as powerful for characterizing the temporal and spatial properties of axons with brain stimulation as the refractory period and collision methods discussed in Chapters 6 and 7. Impatient readers may wish to skip to that material, although the present chapter lays some of the groundwork for the axonal interpretation of those chapters.

EXPONENTIAL MODEL OF LOCAL POTENTIAL

A single, subthreshold stimulating pulse evokes a local potential in cells that outlasts the duration of the pulse. This subthreshold, local potential is measured by placing a recording electrode inside the cell immediately adjacent to a stim-

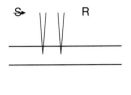

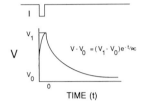

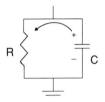

Figure 5-1. Exponential model of local potential. Intracellular stimulation of an axon (above) evokes a fast voltage change, which decays roughly exponentially after the pulse (middle). A perfect exponential results from passing current through a capacitor (below).

ulating electrode. A weak, depolarizing pulse produces a local potential that increases in size during the pulse, then decreases to baseline following the pulse. The peak amplitude of the local potential is roughly proportional to the stimulating current. This potential is called *local* because it does not conduct along the axon without decrement, like an action potential, but decays quickly as a function of distance from the stimulating electrode (Hodgkin, 1938).

The roughly exponential decay of the local potential suggests that below threshold the membrane works like a resistor and capacitor in parallel (Figure 5-1). This circuit charges up exponentially when current pulses are applied and discharges exponentially when the pulses are terminated. The equation for the discharge is $V - V_o = (V_1 - V_o) \, e^{(-t/\tau)}$, where V is the voltage, V_o is the voltage at rest, V_1 is the voltage at the offset of the pulse, t is the time after offset, and τ is the time constant of the circuit. In this circuit, τ equals the resistance times the capacitance.

Local potential summation

Two cathodal pulses, each of which is unable to fire an axon when delivered alone, can sum to produce a single firing when delivered together. The first of these two pulses is called the conditioning (C) pulse, and the second is called the testing (T) pulse, with the time from C pulse onset to T pulse onset called the C-T interval. The local potential due to the C pulse sums with the local potential due to the T pulse. The current of the T pulse required to produce one firing increases as the C-T interval increases, due to the decay of the C pulse local potential. Following the decay of local potential summation, there is sometimes a period, called the depression interval, during which the current of the T pulse must be slightly greater than at rest to produce excitation (Erlanger & Gasser, 1937).

The local potential can be measured indirectly by delivering T pulses at various C-T intervals and testing current thresholds (Tasaki, 1942). When equal-current cathodal pulses are used, the threshold for excitation increases as the C-T interval increases. According to the exponential model: $(I_{sp}/I_{ct}) - 1 = e^{(-t/\tau)}$, where I_{sp} is the current threshold for a single pulse, and I_{ct} is the current threshold at a C T interval of t. The variable t is measured by plotting $(I_{sp}/I_{ct}) - 1$ on semilog paper, since $\log [(I_{sp}/I_{ct}) - 1] = -t/\tau$. If the local potential is exponential, a straight line with slope $-1/\tau$ will be observed on this plot.

Unit data

The data observed following stimulation of single axons do not always agree with the simple exponential model. The first problem is that the membrane is not like a single capacitor, but like many capacitors in parallel (Figure 5-2, top). The exponential model is approximated if these capacitors are charged simultaneously (uniform polarization), as by a wire through the center of an axon. If a microelectrode tip (point polarization) is used, however, the membrane capacitance nearest the tip is charged first, and more distant capacitors are charged later. In this case, the local potential drops more quickly than a simple exponential at first (Jack et al., 1983, pp. 33 and 54–58; Hodgkin & Rushton, 1946; Figure 5-2, bottom, line b). A larger electrode tip or an electrode positioned distant from the axon results in more uniform polarization and a closer approximation to an exponential curve whose time constant is that of the membrane, than a small electrode tip touching or inside the axon.

The second problem is that when the depolarization is just below threshold, the local potential lasts longer and is not close to exponential (line c). The cause of this longer potential is that just below threshold for excitation some Na^+ channels open, but not enough of them to produce an action potential. The size of this "local response" can be measured by comparing the potential following depolarizing stimuli to those following hyperpolarizing stimuli of the same strength (Hodgkin, 1938). Hyperpolarizing stimuli produce a linear increase in voltage with increasing current, but depolarizing stimuli produce a

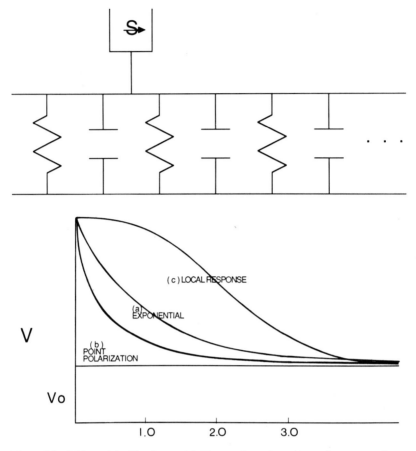

Figure 5-2. Cable model of local potential. The membrane is made up of many capacitances in parallel, so that the local potential does not decay exponentially when the stimulus is applied to a single point. The response following point polarization (b) is more concave than the exponential (a). The local response to channel opening (c), however, is more convex than the exponential.

linear current-voltage relationship only when virtually all channels remain closed. The local response is slight, however, unless the current of the C pulse is very close to threshold (Figure 5-3).

When brain units are stimulated with large or distant extracellular electrodes, local potential summation can be remarkably close to exponential. Figure 5-4A shows 3 midbrain units stimulated by a 200-μm electrode in the MFB. The plot of log (I_{sp}/I_{ct}) -1 versus C-T interval is close to linear. The variable τ was estimated between 0.08 to 0.14 msec and was independent of pulse duration. These estimates may not be exactly the time constants of the membranes for the reasons described above, but should be very close. Local responses are not clearly evident in these data. Very few data have been collected on local poten-

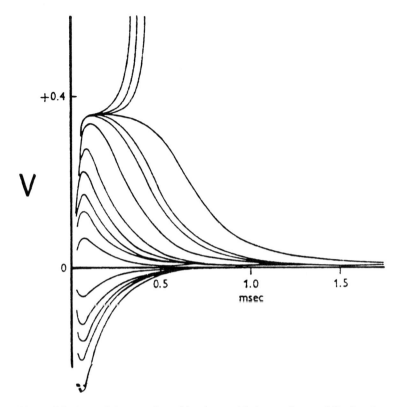

Figure 5-3. Intracellular recording of local potentials in a crab axon following short duration intracellular stimuli (Hodgkin, 1938). The upper six traces were responses to the same intensity stimulus (1.00 threshold), three of which excited the cell and three of which produced long-lasting local potentials. The next six traces were responses to depolarizing stimuli .96, .85, .71, .57, .43 and .21 of the strength of the threshold stimulus, and the bottom five traces are hyperpolarizing stimuli .21, .43, .57, .71, and 1.0 of the strength of the threshold depolarizing stimulus. The voltage scale is expressed as percentage of the 40-mV spike height.

tial summation properties, however, so local potential summation has limited value for characterizing axons at the present time.

STRENGTH-DURATION CURVE

The current required to stimulate an axon with a single pulse decreases as pulse duration increases (Figure 5-5). The minimum current for excitation at long pulse durations is called the rheobase. An estimate of the time of summation, called the chronaxie, is determined by the duration at which the required current is twice rheobase.

Chronaxies of central nervous system (CNS) myelinated axons measured with

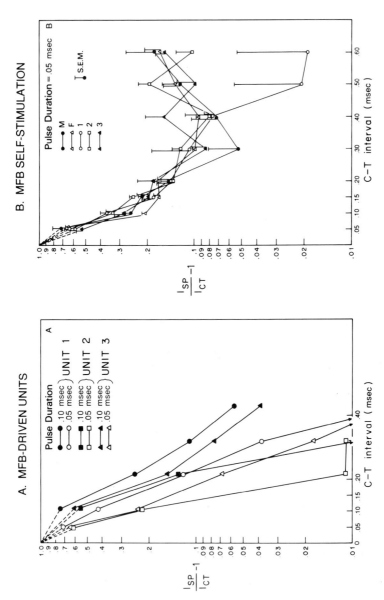

Figure 5-4. Local potential summation in brain stimulation. Left, current via an MFB stimulating electrode required to activate 3 midbrain units recorded extracellularly. Right, current in MFB required to induce a bar-pressing rate of 40 per minute in rats. The ordinate shows current at each C-T interval (Ic-t) compared to single-pulse current (Isp) plotted on log coordinates, so that the curves should be straight lines to fit the exponential model (Yeomans et al., 1979).

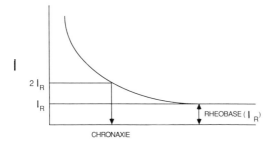

PULSE DURATION

Figure 5-5. Strength-duration curve. The rheobase is the minimum required current at long pulse durations. The chronaxie is the duration at which twice the rheobase current is required.

extracellular stimulation vary from 40 to 260 μsec (Ranck, 1975; Hentall et al., 1984). When measured intracellularly, the values range from 130 to 710 μsec. It is not known why these values are longer (Ranck, 1975). Chronaxies of peripheral axons vary from 29 to 700 μsec, so the range is similar. It is not known what features of axons alter their chronaxies, although it is presumably related to their membrane time constants.

The time of summation measured in the strength-duration experiment is related to the time of local potential summation. For the resistor-capacitor model of Figure 5-1, the strength-duration curve is: $I = Ir/[1 - e^{(D/\tau)}]$, where I is the threshold current. Ir is the rheobase current, and D is the pulse duration. The strength-duration relationship measures the time constant of charging up the circuit, while the local potential summation relationship measures the time constant of discharge of the circuit. These two time constants are equal in the resistor-capacitor model.

Unit data

Strength-duration curves in units often do not fit the exponential equation perfectly, but are fit slightly better by a hyperbolic equation, $I = Ir(1 + c/D)$, where c is the summation time of the hyperbolic equation. These two functions are remarkably similar in shape (Figure 5-6), but when the two functions are fit to the same data, the exponential function is slightly more concave. The hyperbolic equation is empirical, lacking a simple theoretical basis.

The time parameters of exponential and hyperbolic equations can be evaluated by linearizing the data. If $\log [1 - (Ir/I)]$ is plotted versus duration (D), the exponential curve is linear with slope $-1/\tau$, and chronaxie $= .332\ \tau$. If I/Ir is plotted versus $1/D$, the hyperbolic curve is linear with slope equal to the chronaxie (Milner & Laferriere, 1982).

Strength-duration curves may deviate from a simple exponential for at least three reasons. First, point polarization charges the membrane differently than

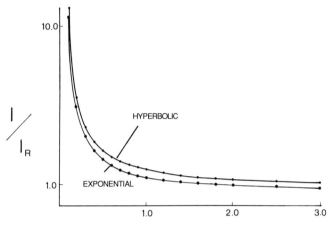

PULSE DURATION

Figure 5-6. The strength-duration curve for the hyperbolic model, $I = Ir\,(1 + C/D)$ is similar to that for the exponential model, $I = Ir/(1 - e^{-D}/\tau)$. The horizontal axis is expressed in units of c or τ.

uniform polarization as discussed above. The time constant of the strength-duration curve is shorter when measured with a small tip electrode close to the axon, than with a large tip or an intraaxonal wire (Noble & Stein, 1966; Fozzard & Schoenberg, 1972; West & Wolstencroft, 1983). In brain stimulation, only neurons very close to a microelectrode are greatly affected by this factor, however.

Second, near-threshold depolarization opens channels, and this alters the form of the strength-duration curve, as previously discussed for local potential summation (Noble & Stein, 1966). In strength-duration curves, long duration pulses produce gradual depolarizations that approach threshold slowly. Therefore, the stimulation is in the near-threshold range for longer periods of time in strength-duration experiments than in local potential summation experiments. This factor can lengthen the time constant of the strength-duration curve.

Third, the axon may accommodate to long duration pulses. Accommodation is observed by an increase in the threshold for excitation following stimulation with long duration cathodal pulses. This increase in threshold shortens the time at which rheobase is reached. Consequently, the rheobase on which time constants and chronaxies are estimated is not a fixed or asymptotic value. Accommodation can either shorten or lengthen the estimated time constant, however (Jack et al., 1983). Accommodation may account for the depression interval in some axons.

Jack et al. (1983) conclude, "In general, therefore, experimentally determined strength-duration curves do not give reliable information on the true membrane time constant." In the conditions relevant to brain stimulation (extracellular electrodes with local, rather than uniform, polarization), the relationship between local potential summation, strength-duration constants, and membrane time constants has not been studied carefully, to my knowledge. In 3 midbrain units, the time constants of strength-duration curves averaged 0.30 msec, while local potential summation time constants averaged 0.10 msec (Matthews, 1977; Yeomans et al., 1979), but the membrane time constant was not measured intracellularly. The local potential summation method seems preferable because it is less affected by accommodation. Furthermore, the effects of subthreshold channel openings can be measured by comparing the effects of hyperpolarizing and depolarizing C pulses.

Multiple firings to long duration pulses

When pulse durations longer than the absolute refractory period are used, more than one firing can occur in response to a single long-duration pulse. If accommodation is strong, however, these multiple firings are eliminated or restricted to the first part of the stimulating pulse. Many different types of multiple firings to single pulses occur, and no single model can be applied to all cases (Jack et al., 1983, Chapter 11).

BEHAVIORAL STUDIES OF LOCAL POTENTIAL SUMMATION

Local potential summation can be measured behaviorally by comparing the required current at each C-T interval (I_{ct}) to the required current in the single pulse condition (I_{sp}). In Figure 5-4B, log $[(I_{sp}/I_{ct}) - 1]$ is plotted as a function of C-T interval, so that the behavioral data can be compared to the unit data of Figure 5-4A. Each curve represents tests via a single electrode. The variability between electrodes was slight at C-T intervals below 0.4 msec. The decline at C-T intervals from 0.1 to 0.3 msec was similar to that observed in midbrain units driven by MFB electrodes (Figure 5-4A). In the self-stimulation data, the time constant was near 0.10 msec, but the curves bowed upward slightly. This bowing might be expected when averaging over units with different time constants. The rise at C-T intervals from 0.4 to 0.6 msec is due to recovery from refractoriness (Chapter 6).

To test the hypothesis that near-threshold depolarization alters the form of the behavioral data, anodal C pulses were delivered to hyperpolarize the axons. In this case, the T pulses must be higher in current to compensate for the local hyperpolarization of the anodal pulses. The data were not significantly different from the cathodal data except at C-T intervals above 0.4 msec. (The data are plotted on linear coordinates to show the negative values at these longer C-T intervals.) Since hyperpolarization does not open Na^+ channels, this result suggests that ''local responses'' account for little in the behavioral data (Figure 5-7), which is consistent with the unit data above showing little evidence of a local response.

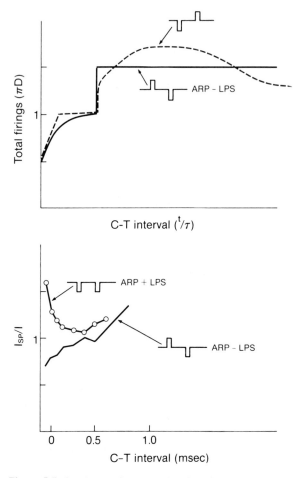

Figure 5-7. Local potential summation for MFB self-stimulation when anodal C pulses are delivered. The current of the C pulses was constant and the current of the T pulses varied until the response criterion was achieved (Yeomans et al., 1979). See Appendix I for further discussion.

In behavioral experiments where many neurons must be stimulated, it is important to hold the field of axons constant, so that the results do not depend on the location of the substrates around the electrode. If current is held constant and frequency is varied, however, the number of axons excited increases with pulse duration in the strength-duration experiment, or decreases with C-T interval in the local potential summation experiment. A better way to measure subthreshold summation is to vary the current, at a constant frequency. If all axons have the same summation time, the same axons are excited in all summation conditions.

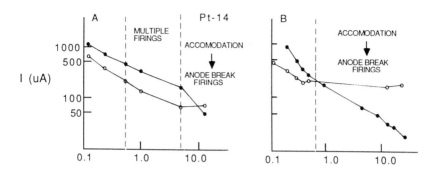

PULSE DURATION (MSEC)

Figure 5-8. Strength-duration curves for MFB self-stimulation (after Matthews, 1977). Solid circles, anodal pulses; open circles, cathodal pulses. The proposed interpretation ("multiple and anodal-break firings") is discussed in the text.

BEHAVIORAL STUDIES OF STRENGTH-DURATION CURVES

Strength-duration curves obtained for MFB self-stimulation have the same general form as unit strength-duration curves: increases in pulse duration result in decreases in the current required (Szabo & Milner, 1973; White, 1976; Matthews, 1977; Barry et al., 1974; Ward, 1959; Milner & Laferriere, 1982). The chronaxies, however, range from 0.5 to 3.0 msec, which are much longer than the 0.1 to 0.6 msec chronaxies observed in units driven by the same electrodes. The unit data reach rheobase at 1.0 msec, but the behaviorally derived curves continue to decline at durations from 1 to 5 msec (Matthews, 1977, 1978) (Figure 5-8, left panel, dashed lines).

Furthermore, these behavioral curves cannot be fit by either hyperbolic or exponential equations; the behavioral data drop even slower than the hyperbolic curve. By contrast, unit data generally fall in between hyperbolic and exponential curves, often fitting one or the other curve better.

Multiple firings

The decrease in required current using long duration pulses in the behavioral curves may be caused by multiple firings (Matthews, 1978). Multiple firings can be a serious problem in behavioral experiments, since axons near the electrode can be stimulated by current densities many times threshold. This means that each 5-msec pulse may produce several firings in a single axon. The summation that occurs following multiple firings is not in the axons at the stimulation site but in subsequent synapses, and is therefore unrelated to the local membrane time constant. Consequently, the rheobase in behavioral strength-duration curves is even more suspect than in unit curves.

Because of this problem, it has been suggested that summation time estimates should be based only on short duration pulses (White, 1976; Hentall et al., 1984). A true rheobase cannot be estimated, and so τ or c estimates must be based on curve fitting. Estimates of τ based on fits to the first 0.4 msec of these truncated strength-duration curves are 0.15 msec for MFB self-stimulation (Milner & Laferriere, 1982), which is similar to estimates of τ derived from units driven by MFB stimulation (Matthews, 1978). Hentall et al. (1984) estimated τ at 0.18 msec for the analgesic effects of medulla stimulation, which is similar to the 0.10 and 0.18 estimates of τ they obtained in two units driven by medulla stimulation. Therefore, behavioral estimates of unit strength-duration properties are safest when based on the first half-msec of the behaviorally measured strength-duration curve.

Accommodation

Measuring accommodation is important for two reasons. First, accommodation occurs in a few tenths of a millisecond in some axons and not for tens of milliseconds in other axons, so accommodation is a powerful characteristic for differentiating axons. Second, accommodation alters the strength-duration curve at long durations and blocks multiple firings. Therefore, the interpretation of strength-duration curves at long pulse durations requires a measure of accommodation.

Matthews (1977) proposed that accommodation can be measured by comparing anodal strength-duration curves to cathodal strength-duration curves. When anodal pulses are used, excitation can occur at pulse onset ("anode-make") or at pulse offset ("anode-break"). Anode-make excitation is due to depolarization of distant nodes (Chapter 2). Anode-break excitation, however, is due to the local depolarization that occurs following a hyperpolarizing pulse. If accommodation occurs to a long duration hyperpolarizing pulse, the depolarization at pulse offset can excite the axon. Consequently, the strength of accommodation can be measured by comparing the current threshold for anodal and cathodal pulses of long duration. If accommodation occurs, the threshold for long anodal pulses will drop relative to the thresholds for long cathodal pulses.

Figure 5-8 shows the relationship between anodal and cathodal strength-duration curves observed for two different responses—MFB self-stimulation on the left panel and a motor response to the same stimulation on the right panel. The results for the two responses were very different, suggesting that different types of neurons mediate the two responses. The different results obtained for the two behaviors cannot be attributed to the electrode or electrode-tissue interface, since the same electrode was used for both sets of data.

At durations shorter than 0.5 msec, the anodal and cathodal curves were roughly parallel on the log–log plot, suggesting that the ratio between cathode- and anode-make excitation stays roughly constant. For self-stimulation this ratio was always close to 2:1, but for the motor response the ratio was usually 3:1 or 4:1 (Matthews, 1977). It is not clear whether this difference reflects differences in myelination or the geometrical relationship between electrode and substrate, or other factors.

At longer durations, the thresholds for anodal strength-duration curves decreased sharply, suggesting that accommodation occurred. Accommodation apparently occurred sooner and was stronger for the motor response than for self-stimulation. To support this idea, Matthews showed that the motor response always occurred 20 msec after pulse *onset* for short duration anodal pulses, but always occurred 20 msec after pulse *offset* for long duration anodal pulses. Anode-break firing, therefore, accounts for the decline in threshold for long duration anodal pulses. There must be multiple firings at anodal break, however, since current threshold decreased to one-tenth at durations longer than the cathodal rheobase, and anodal stimulation became more effective than cathodal stimulation.

Since accommodation blocks multiple firings, the hypothesis that multiple firings account for the decline in cathodal curves at long pulse durations is also supported by Matthews' data. As soon as accommodation is evident in anodal curves, the cathodal curves stop their decline. This is clear because the cathodal curves stop their decline before 1 msec in the motor response data, but not until 5 msec in the self-stimulation data.

The anodal strength-duration curve, then, adds much information to the cathodal curve. The anode–cathode ratio can be determined at short durations. The strength of accommodation can be assessed at longer durations. From this, the possible contribution of cathodal multiple firings can be roughly evaluated. More work on anodal strength-duration curves is needed. These experiments are technically difficult, however, due to the problems of anodal lesions (Appendix II). Large surface-area platinum electrodes should be used to prevent metal ion deposits, and short pulse durations should be tried before attempting longer pulse durations.

CONCLUSIONS

Local potential summation is measured by comparing the required current at each C-T interval to the required current using single pulses. Unit and behavioral local potential summation curves obtained for MFB self-stimulation are roughly exponential with a time constant on the order of 0.1 msec. This estimate may be close to the membrane time constant. Anodal C pulses did not measurably alter the shape of curves for MFB self-stimulation, which suggests that local channel openings did not appreciably alter the results.

Strength-duration curves are measured by the required current at different pulse durations. Unit strength-duration curves yield longer time constants than local potential summation curves. Behaviorally measured strength-duration curves for MFB self-stimulation drop even slower than hyperbolic curves and yield much longer chronaxies than unit curves. If only pulse durations shorter than

0.4 msec are considered, however, the curves have time constants similar to unit strength-duration curves. At pulse durations longer than 0.4 msec, multiple firings in axons near the electrode appear to cause the steady decline in these behavioral curves.

Accommodation can be measured by the decline in anodal strength-duration curves as compared with cathodal curves. Accommodation prevents cathodal excitation, especially multiple firings. The amount of accommodation or multiple firings can vary considerably in different systems, and so anodal strength-duration curves may prove to be a powerful way to characterize neural systems using brain summation.

The challenge for brain stimulation is to characterize populations of neurons, even when these neurons have different excitability properties. Temporal summation curves average the excitability curves of many neurons, and so the different summation times of the constituent axons or synaptic integrators cannot be adequately extracted in behavioral experiments.

POSTAXONAL SUMMATION

Pulses that are delivered more than a msec apart do not sum in axons, due to the short axon time constants. The temporal summation that occurs following spaced pulses must be due to summation of action potentials in postsynaptic cells. These pulses can be presented as two pulses, or two pulse trains (akin to the local potential summation experiment), or as a continuous train (akin to the strength-duration experiment).

The model for synaptic summation in the central nervous system is the monosynaptic stretch reflex (Eccles, 1964). Eccles and colleagues were the first to put microelectrodes inside central nervous system cells. This technical innovation was rewarded by the discovery that inside cells are novel potentials activated by synaptic inputs. They called these *postsynaptic potentials* (PSPs). The PSPs are graded and quasi-exponential, like the local potentials first observed in axons by Hodgkin, but have time constants at least an order of magnitude longer, due to the larger membrane area of cells. Also PSPs can be activated by peripheral stimulation rather than local electrical stimulation.

Figure 5-9 shows some of the first intracellular PSPs recorded by Eccles's group. Stretching of a muscle was known to powerfully excite a reflexive contraction of the same muscle via a fast spinal reflex. Opposing muscles are inhibited. Activation of stretch receptors initiates action potentials in sensory neurons, which, in turn, initiate a large *excitatory postsynaptic potential* (EPSP) in ventral horn motor neurons (Figure 5-9). The EPSP rises quickly, then decays almost exponentially with a time constant that ranges from 3 to 6 msec in cat hindlimb motor neurons. The fixed, short latency of the response makes it clear that only one synapse can intervene between sensory and motor neurons.

Furthermore, the properties of synaptic summation in the spinal cord, first described by Sherrington (1906), are explained by the properties of summation of PSPs. The height of the EPSP increases as the number of afferents excited

EPSP-
SPATIAL
SUMMATION

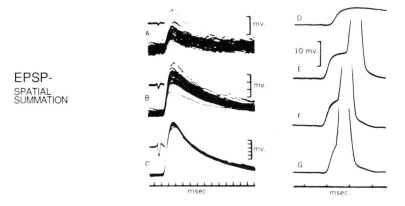

REFLEX-
TEMPORAL
SUMMATION

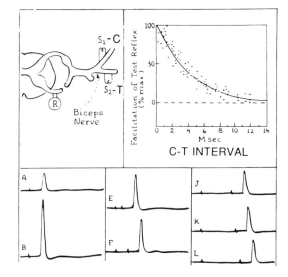

Figure 5-9. Summation in the monosynaptic stretch reflex. Above, EPSPs recorded by electrodes inside cat lumbar motoneurons. The size of the EPSP increased with the current of sensory nerve activation (A-C). The dorsal root potential (inset to the upper left of each record) shows that the increased size of the EPSP is related to the increased number of axons activated. The latency of the action potential also decreased (D-G; Eccles, 1964). Below, temporal summation due to stimulation of two sensory nerves. The size of the ventral root potential is larger at short C-T intervals than at long C-T intervals (Lloyd, 1946). No refractory period was observed because separate nerves were stimulated. Bottom: A, the response to a single pulse, B-L, the responses to two pulses at increasing C-T intervals. These data are plotted along with other tests in the graph immediately above.

87

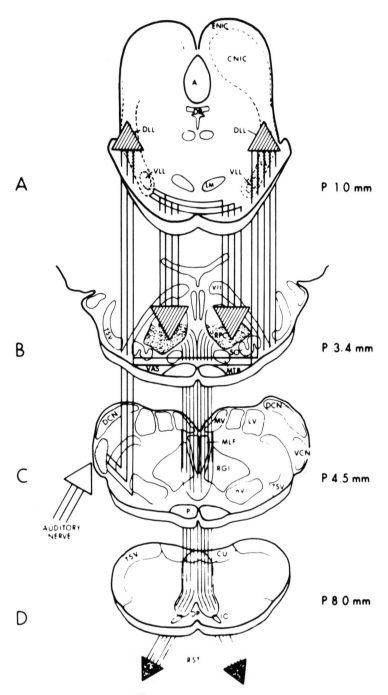

Figure 5-10. Startle reflexes evoked by tones and electrical brain stimulation. A. Davis' (1984) model of the primary acoustic startle reflex circuit. B. The latency of the response (measured by hindlimb EMG) decreased as the placement of the electrode advanced through the circuit from the cochlear nucleus to the spinal cord, proceeding from the bottom line to the top line.

88

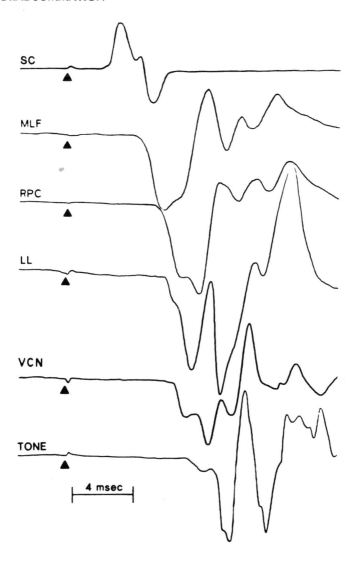

increases (spatial summation). Temporal summation occurs due to the overlap of EPSPs: if the EPSPs overlap, the summed potential is larger and the probability of a motor neuron action potential (and muscle twitch) is higher. Therefore, the properties of the EPSP account for the properties of spatial and temporal summation found for the stretch reflex.

Temporal summation in the startle reflex circuit

A loud, sharp noise evokes in mammals a startle reflex. This is a rapid protective response of many muscles, including eye closure, shoulder hunching, and hindlimb extension. Following acoustic stimulation, the latency of the hindlimb response in rats is only 8 msec. Unlike most reflexes, this acoustic startle reflex activates both flexors and extensors.

The startle reflex is mediated by a simple brain stem circuit. A startle-like response can be evoked by a single electrical pulse in any of several auditory and brainstem areas (Davis et al., 1982). The latency of the hindlimb response is 6.5 msec following cochlear nucleus stimulation, 5 msec following reticular formation stimulation, and 3 msec following spinal cord stimulation. Lesions of any of these structures block the acoustic startle reflex (Davis et al., 1982). These results suggest that a serial circuit passing through these brain stem sites mediates startle with a minimum of 3–5 synapses in the circuit (Figure 5-10).

The axons in the startle circuit leaving brain stem for spinal cord are believed to be large, fast reticulospinal axons. Stimulation of homologous sites in cats activates spinal hindlimb motor neurons (both flexors and extensors) monosynaptically (Grillner & Lund, 1968; Peterson et al., 1979).

If a second stimulating pulse is delivered, the current required for a fixed startle response is reduced at a C-T interval of 2 msec, then rises rapidly with a mean time constant of 4 msec. The time constant of summation in the startle reflex induced by brain stimulation, then, is almost the same as the time constant of the monosynaptic EPSP recorded from the spinal hindlimb motor neurons (Figure 5-11). This suggests that the startle reflex is monosynaptic from brainstem reticular formation to spinal motor neurons.

When the stimulus is delivered to the cochlear nucleus, the time course of temporal summation is slower (although still quite fast). This suggests that the synapses between cochlear nucleus and reticular formation alter the temporal relationship between the evoked action potentials.

This two-pulse brain stimulation experiment, then, is like the local potential summation experiment described above—a trade-off between C-T interval and current. The process is again exponential, but the time constant of synaptic summation is 40 times longer than axonal summation. Both processes result from summation of subthreshold, graded potentials with fast rise times and exponential decay.

Double-pulse tests of summation in other systems

In motor cortex, two-pulse stimulation of forelimb responses in rats produces an effect like the startle reflex, only the summation is slower (Yeomans &

Figure 5-11. Upper, paired-pulse stimulation of "startle" responses from the caudal reticular formation in rats (Yeomans et al., 1989). Temporal summation (measured by the current thresholds for a constant startle response) declined with almost the same time course as the monosynaptic reticulospinal EPSP below. Lower, spike-averaged EPSPs recorded from four cat lumbar motoneurons. The stimulating electrode was in the medial longitudinal fasciculus of the medulla shown by the arrow above. The EPSPs appear to be monosynaptically driven by medullary stimulation (Peterson et al., 1979).

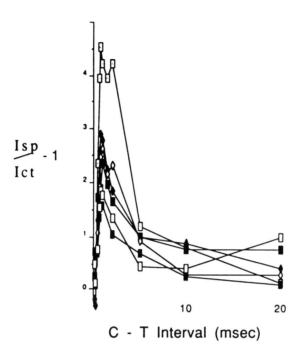

$$\frac{Isp}{Ict} - 1$$

C - T Interval (msec)

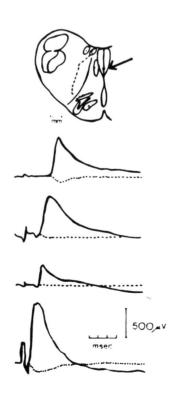

500 µV

msec

Chapman, 1989). For most systems, however, more than two pulses are required to produce observable behavior. Consequently, the EPSPs must overlap considerably to produce temporal summation. When trains of pulses are delivered, the shape of the unitary EPSP is hard to determine from threshold changes, unlike the local potential summation experiment, where the unitary local potential can be approximated by the rapid decay in threshold within the first half msec. In most experiments using paired-pulse trains, little effect of C-T interval has been found that is clearly attributable to synaptic summation (see Chapter 6).

A related way to test integration is by delivering two trains of pulses. Deutsch and Collins (1965) showed that the required current for MFB self-stimulation increases as the interval between trains increases from 100 to 400 msec. The mechanism for this long integration time is not clear.

Current versus train duration measures of summation

A more generally applicable procedure is to measure the trade-off between current and train duration. This procedure is the synaptic analog of the strength-duration experiment. For the startle reflex, summation is very rapid and so the minimum current (rheobase) is reached in 20 msec, yielding a synaptic ''chronaxie'' of about 8 msec (Figure 5-12). For MFB self-stimulation, the minimum current is reached in about 2 seconds, yielding a ''chronaxie'' for self-stimulation of about 450 msec (Gallistel, 1978). Estimating the form of the underlying EPSP from such data is quite problematic, however, requiring several strong assumptions (Gallistel, 1973; Norman & Gallistel, 1978). The strength-duration method is useful, since it can be applied to all systems and yields large differences between systems.

In this experiment, either current (spatial summation) or frequency (temporal summation) can be traded off against train duration in most systems. When many pulses are required for a response, it is preferable to measure temporal summation by varying frequency and holding current constant in order to hold the field of stimulated axons constant. To measure spatial summation, the current can be varied, but it is difficult to determine whether the changes are due to changes in synaptic summation or to changes in the density of axons in the varying field of excitation. A stronger but more difficult method of measuring spatial summation is discussed in Chapter 7, using two stimulating electrodes and comparing frequency thresholds.

Is summation linear over time?

A maintained train of pulses can produce a steady output, or an increased or decreased response. For example, the cumulative number of circles to a maintained train of stimulating pulses is shown in Figure 5-13. Stimulation of the pons resulted in circling at a nearly constant rate for 90 seconds after the initial start up in the first seconds. Stimulation of the frontal cortex at the same frequency resulted in circling that gradually slowed within 10–40 seconds.

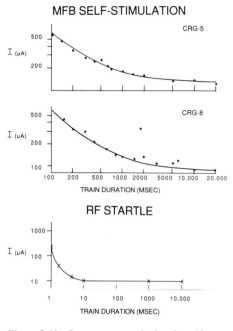

Figure 5-12. Current versus train duration. Above, summation in two MFB self-stimulation sites (Gallistel et al., 1981). Below, summation in reticular formation sites evoking "startle".

Many synaptic factors can account for these temporal properties. The synapses can be plastic, showing facilitation or antifacilitation. The time constant of the cell body can be short or long, to produce short or long EPSPs. Long EPSPs can produce multiple firings or accommodation at the initial segments. Inhibitory feedback loops can disrupt the pattern of excitation. These factors can make a continuous train of presynaptic pulses into a highly variable stimulus in postsynaptic axons. These alterations can occur at each synapse throughout a system.

Consequently, the temporal summation characteristics of a system cannot clearly define the mechanisms which cause that response. Especially, procedures for determining whether the first synapses, first initial segments, or subsequent stages produce the temporal alteration have not been devised. Temporal summation, then, is more of a descriptive science than an analytical one at the present time.

Conclusions

Temporal summation of action potentials in the postaxonal circuits leading to behavior can be measured by delivering trains of short-duration pulses. These summation times are peculiar to each system, and vary from summation for

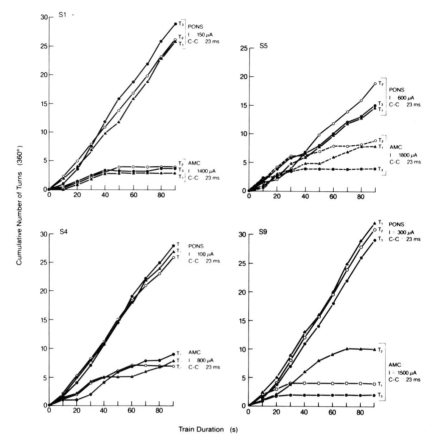

Figure 5-13. Circling in pontine sites is steady for 90 seconds of stimulation. Circling in antero-medial cortex sites is less reliable and usually stops within 30 seconds (Tehovnik & Yeomans, 1987).

only a few milliseconds to summation over many seconds. The mechanisms of summation are poorly understood except in monosynaptic circuits, where the form of the summation can be nearly exponential, mimicking the form of the postsynaptic potential.

FURTHER READINGS

Jack, J.J.B., Noble, D., & Tsien, R.W. *Electric Current Flow in Excitable Cells.* London: Oxford University Press, 1983. Reviews excitation of nerve and muscle, including mathematical models.

Hodgkin, A.L., & Rushton, W.A.H. The electrical constants of a crustacean nerve fibre. *Proceedings of the Royal Society (London),* 1946, *B133,* 444–479. This empirical paper describes the passive electrical properties of unmyelinated axons.

6

Refractory Periods

Paired-pulse stimulation is the most powerful method for characterizing the temporal properties of axon bundles. In this chapter, paired-pulse stimulation is delivered through a single electrode to measure the refractory periods of single axons or of axon bundles mediating electrically evoked behaviors. The quantitative methods used to estimate absolute refractory period distributions, and the assumptions of the refractory period model are discussed. The refractory period experiment is the foundation for the collision and current–distance experiments discussed in Chapter 7.

REFRACTORY PERIODS

The recovery of excitable cells following stimulation consists of an absolute refractory period (ARP), a relative refractory period (RRP), and often a supernormal period (SNP) and subnormal period (SubNP). Each of these periods can be separately measured in behavioral experiments, so I begin with a short review of the physiology of these events.

When an above-threshold C pulse is delivered, an axon is absolutely inexcitable by T pulses for a time period called the ARP (Figure 6-1). The duration of the ARP is roughly the duration of the action potential (Paintal, 1978). An RRP follows in which the axon can be excited, but only by currents greater than those required at rest. Following the RRP, an SNP and a SubNP are often, but not always, found. The series of threshold changes following excitation is called the *poststimulation excitability cycle*. Unlike local potential summation, this cycle is relatively independent of the intensity of the C pulse (Raymond & Lettvin, 1978).

The refractory period is generally measured by a recording electrode distant from the stimulation site. With this method, the initiation of action potentials at the stimulation site is not observed, but rather the conduction of action potentials to the recording electrode. In some cases, it has been shown that firings near the stimulating electrode fail to conduct. Consequently, the *refractory period* observed at a distance is more accurately called the *minimum C-T interval for which two action potentials are measured at the recording electrode* (Paintal, 1978); however, the term *refractory period* will be used here in all cases.

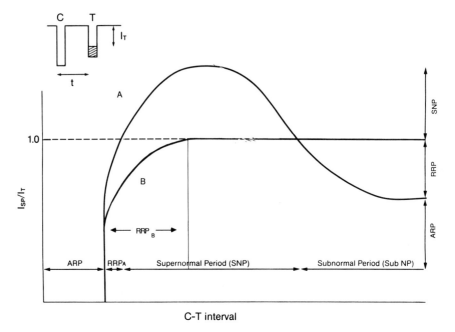

Figure 6-1. Poststimulation excitability cycle. An above-threshold conditioning pulse is followed by a variable intensity testing pulse. The T-pulse current required to evoke a second action potential is measured at each C-T interval. The excitability at each C-T interval is measured by the required current at rest (I_{sp}) divided by the required T pulse current (I_t). In some cases, large supernormal and subnormal periods may be observed (A). In other cases, supernormal and subnormal periods are absent, but the relative refractory period is long (B).

Similarly, refractory periods measured by behavioral trade off data are more correctly called *C-T intervals for which the frequency required for responding decreases.*

Refractoriness is due to the fact that sodium channels remain open for a short period of time and therefore cannot initiate a second action potential until they are closed again. Recovery occurs when many channels close and are then available to be reopened. Although the duration of opening of single Na$^+$ channels is variable, the duration of the ARP is relatively fixed for a single axon, since it is linked to the mean duration of channel opening. The ARP can be increased, however, if the axon is stimulated at very high rates that approach the maximum rate at which the axon can fire.

The ARPs of different axons vary from 0.3 to more than 5 msec. In general, fast-conducting fibers have shorter ARPs than slow-conducting fibers (Hursch, 1939). The relationship between ARP and conduction velocity is almost identical in peripheral (Hursch, 1939; Paintal, 1978) or central axons (Swadlow & Waxman, 1978; Figure 6-2). The correlation between ARP and fiber diameter, however, is not as strong as between conduction velocity and fiber diameter.

The RRP corresponds to the time when many, but not all, of the Na$^+$ channels are closed and ready to be reopened. The duration of the RRP depends

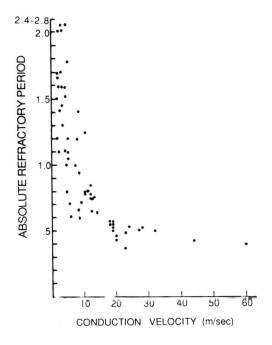

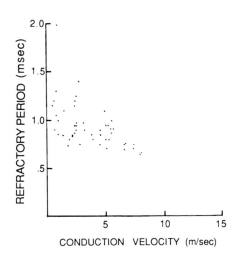

Figure 6-2. Absolute refractory period versus conduction velocity. Each point represents recordings from a single unit. Upper panel, peripheral nerve axons (After Hursch, 1939, and Paintal, 1978). Lower panel, callosal axons (Swadlow & Waxman, 1978).

strongly on whether an SNP occurs or not. When no SNP is evident, the RRP is prolonged as recovery proceeds asymptotically to the resting current threshold (Figure 6-1, line B). When an SNP occurs, however, the RRP is short, because the current threshold drops quickly below the resting threshold (Figure 6-1, line A; Graham, 1934). The duration of the SNP period, in turn, depends on the onset of the SubNP.

SUPERNORMAL AND SUBNORMAL PERIODS

SNPs and SubNPs are highly variable. After a single stimulation, the SNP is usually less than 30 percent, and the SubNP less than 10 percent, in large myelinated axons (Erlanger & Gasser, 1937). When the axon has been stimulated repeatedly, however, both SNPs and SubNPs are stronger and occur sooner (Graham, 1934; Swadlow & Waxman, 1978; Raymond & Lettvin, 1978). As few as five pulses in one second can double the size of the SNP and start a clearly observable SubNP. SNPs and SubNPs can be stronger in slow-conducting fibers than in fast-conducting fibers (Swadlow & Waxman, 1978).

The mechanisms of the SNP and SubNP are still being investigated. In some small myelinated axons, the SNP is related to a slow depolarization following a single action potential, which leaves the axon close to threshold after the Na^+ channels have recovered (Bowe et al., 1985). The source of this depolarizing afterpotential may be a large capacitance under the myelin sheath (Barrett & Barrett, 1982).

When many firings occur, however, repeated channel openings allow K^+ to leave the cell and Na^+ to enter the cell. In this case, the SNP can be due to a transient increase in extracellular K^+, which makes the K^+ equilibrium potential less negative and lowers the threshold for excitation (Eng & Kocsis, 1985). The SubNP is proposed to be due to a slower or longer-lasting increase in intracellular Na^+, which reduces the local equilibrium potential for sodium and raises the threshold for excitation. The action of the sodium-potassium pump and diffusion would reverse both effects (Raymond & Lettvin, 1978; Swadlow et al., 1980).

FREQUENCY FOLLOWING AND AXON TERMINAL FAILURE

A refractory period experiment measures the ability of the axon to fire twice using two pulses. When three or more pulses are delivered, the pulses must be spaced by more than the ARP to fire action potentials following each pulse. Consequently, the frequency that produces one-for-one firing of action potentials following each pulse decreases as the number of pulses increases. This *following frequency* is much less than the reciprocal of the ARP when more than two pulses are delivered (Paintal, 1978).

The failure of axons to conduct high-frequency action potentials can also occur in the fine terminal branches. Smaller axons conduct high-frequency action potentials poorly because these small axons have longer refractory periods and slower conduction velocities (Swadlow et al., 1980). In addition, less post-synaptic excitation can result per firing when presynaptic action potentials are closely spaced in time (Raymond & Lettvin, 1978). This mechanism can reduce the postsynaptic effect of high frequencies.

BEHAVIORAL STUDIES OF REFRACTORY PERIODS

Deutsch (1964) proposed that paired-pulse brain stimulation could be used to measure the refractory periods of the directly excited neurons mediating MFB self-stimulation. Bar-pressing rates were found to increase sharply at C-T intervals near 1.0 msec.

More reliable results were obtained using trade-off data instead of bar-pressing rates. The current or frequency required to produce a constant bar-pressing rate was found to decrease as the C-T interval increased from 0.4 to 1.2 msec (Hu & Coons, 1975; Yeomans & Davis, 1975; Yeomans, 1975).

The trade-off between C-T interval and frequency (Figure 6-3, top) is the most useful. As the C-T interval increases, the frequency of pulse pairs required to produce a constant output decreases. When all axons have recovered from refractoriness, twice as many firings occur, so half as many pulse pairs are needed. The percent recovery is measured by the ratio: $E = (F_{sp}/F_{ct}) - 1$, where F_{sp} is the frequency of pulses required when only C pulses are presented (the single-pulse condition), and F_{ct} is the frequency of pulse pairs required at a given C-T interval. This ratio measures the effectiveness (E) of the T pulses in producing behavior relative to the C pulses.

E is shown in Figure 6-3 for self-stimulation via MFB electrodes. The effectiveness declined rapidly at C-T intervals below 0.4 msec, then rose steadily from 0.4 to 1.2 msec. A gradual rise at longer C-T intervals occurred as well.

The interpretation given to this curve is that the decline in E at C-T intervals below 0.4 msec is due to declining local potential summation, and the rise at C-T intervals above 0.4 msec is due to recovery from refractoriness in the directly stimulated axons producing self-stimulation. Based on this interpretation, "refractory periods" of axons mediating a wide variety of behaviors have been measured.

To take two extreme examples, self-stimulation of the medial prefrontal cortex recovers at C-T intervals of 1.0 to 5.0 msec with the 50 percent point reached above 2.0 msec (Schenk & Shizgal, 1982). By contrast, startle responses evoked by reticular formation stimulation recover at C-T intervals from 0.3 to 0.8 msec, with over half the rise in E occurring from 0.3 to 0.5 msec (Yeomans et al., 1989).

Unit recording

The most direct evidence for the idea that these curves are related to the refractory periods of axons driven from these sites is unit recording data. The distri-

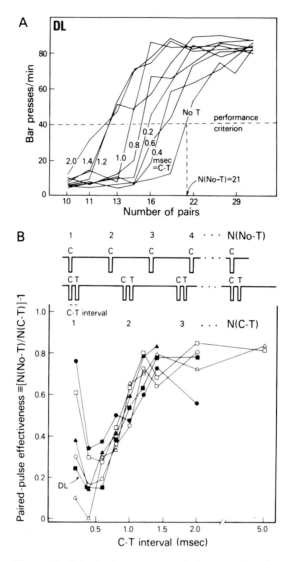

Figure 6-3. Behavioral measurement of refractory periods for
MFB self-stimulation. Upper panel: the number of bar presses
per minute increased with frequency (number) of pairs in a
500-msec train. As the C-T interval increased, the required
frequency decreased. The effectiveness of the T pulses is measured by the leftward shift in the frequency required to reach
the performance criterion. Lower panel: the effectiveness of
the T pulses is shown as a function of C-T interval for six
MFB electrodes (including DL above). After a sharp drop as
C-T interval increased from 0.2 to 0.4 msec, effectiveness rose
steadily from 0.4 to 1.2 msec (After Yeomans, 1975).

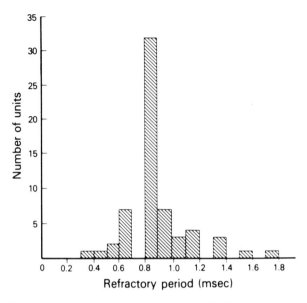

Figure 6-4. Absolute refractory periods of units directly driven by MFB stimulation (Gallistel, 1983, after Rolls, 1974).

bution of ARPs taken from stimulation sites in the MFB are very similar to the behaviorally measured refractory periods for self-stimulation (Figure 6-4).

Although the behavior-producing neurons must have refractory periods included within those of the stimulated neurons, recording data alone cannot prove that the recorded units are responsible for the behavior. Consequently, the strongest evidence for the refractory period interpretation must come from behavioral data that test the parametric properties of this system to determine whether axonal refractory periods account for the complete pattern of results. The following tests of the refractory period hypothesis not only support the hypothesis, but provide further information about MFB self-stimulation.

Effects of frequency

If the rise in E is due to recovery from axonal refractoriness, the results should be relatively insensitive to the frequency of stimulation. If the rise in E is due to axon terminal failure or synaptic effects, the rise might be more sensitive. Hawkins et al. (1983) tested this idea in a Y maze, where rats had a choice between an alley with a 1-second train of single pulses, or an alley with a 1-second train of paired pulses. This choice paradigm tests preference rather than simply self-stimulation rate and so is a better test of the reward value of the stimulation. The baseline frequency in the single-pulse alley was set at 25, 50, 100, or 200 Hz. The frequency of paired pulses was adjusted at each C-T interval until the animal chose the two alleys equally.

The results plotting E versus C-T interval at frequencies from 25 to 200 Hz were almost identical. Therefore, the results do not depend on the particular frequency chosen. Furthermore, the E values at each C-T interval were almost identical to the self-stimulation data of Figure 6-3, suggesting that the same type of axons mediate preference for MFB brain stimulation reward as mediate MFB self-stimulation. Other studies suggest that increases in the frequency above 400 Hz alter the time of recovery, perhaps due to the inability of these MFB axons to follow this frequency.

Absolute refractory periods

If the rise in excitability from 0.4 msec to 1.2 msec is due to recovery from refractoriness, then the curves should be altered by using unequal-current C and T pulses, which change the relative contributions of the ARPs, RRPs, SNPs, and SubNPs. This method of isolating the behavioral effects of each of these periods requires a description of the effects of equal- and unequal-current pulses on a bundle of axons.

Equal-current C and T pulses

Each C pulse activates a population of axons around the electrode tip (Figure 6-5). Those axons nearest the tip are exposed to the highest current densities. If the T pulse is the same current as the C pulse, the axons nearest the tip are exposed to current densities considerably above their resting thresholds. The T pulses, then, will excite all axons near the tip at all C-T intervals longer than their ARPs.

Axons near the edge of the field excited by the C pulse are exposed to current densities barely above their resting thresholds, however. These axons, then, are not stimulated until they recover from their RRPs. Axons not excited by the C pulse can be excited only by local potential summation when T pulses are delivered at very short C-T intervals. These fields are shown in Figure 6-5A for a bundle of axons with identical thresholds. (For details, see Appendix I.)

No new axons can be excited during the SNP using equal-current C and T pulses. To show the SNP, the C pulse must be above threshold, while the T pulse must be below resting threshold for the axon, which cannot occur when the pulses are the same height. Consequently, the SNP is cut off using equal-current C and T pulses. At longer C-T intervals, the SubNP can remove firings in axons barely excited by the C pulse. These are the same axons that show the RRP.

Higher-current T pulse

When the T pulse is much larger than the C pulse, all axons excited by the C pulse are exposed to a current density considerably above their resting thresholds. The T pulse is strong enough, then, to excite all of these axons as soon as they have recovered from their ARPs. In addition, outside this region, the

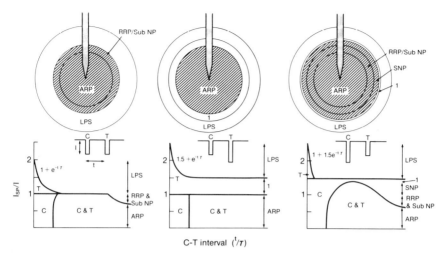

C-T interval ($^t/\tau$)

Figure 6-5. Equal and unequal current C and T pulses (after Yeomans, 1979). Upper drawings show a model of the fields of excitation around a stimulating electrode placed in a homogeneous bundle of like-threshold axons. Nearest the electrode tip, axons recover as soon as their absolute refractory periods (ARPs) are over. Relative refractory period (RRP), supernormal period (SNP), subnormal period (SubNP) and local potential summation (LPS) regions are also shown. Left, equal current C and T pulses; middle, T pulses 1.5 times larger than C pulses; right, C pulses 1.5 times larger than T pulses. Below, excitability curves are shown based on the excitability cycle A shown in Figure 6-1. The variable t is the C-T interval and tau is the time constant of the local potential. The letters C, T, and C & T show which pulse evokes an action potential in each region. The relationship $I = Kr^2$ was used to determine the radii of the fields of excitation.

larger T pulse excites new axons, but these axons are excited at all C-T intervals. Finally, in axons more distant from the electrode, local potential summation occurs at very short C-T interval. The poststimulation excitability cycle is therefore reduced to a step function, with the step at the ARP, for all axons excited by the C pulse (Figure 6-5B).

A higher-current T pulse, then, erases the effects of RRPs, and by a similar argument erases the effects of SNPs and SubNPs. By comparing the higher-current T pulse condition to the equal-current pulses condition, the effects of both RRPs and SubNPs can be measured. In addition, the depression interval may be seen using a larger T pulse, but not using equal-current pulses. These effects are discussed more quantitatively in Appendix I.

Higher-current C pulse

When the C pulse is larger than the T pulse, the field excited by the C pulse is larger (Figure 6-5C). Those axons nearest the electrode fire a second time immediately after the ARP. Axons farther from the electrode fire later in the RRP, as in the equal-current pulses condition. Axons added by the larger C pulse are excited during their SNPs by the weaker T pulse. A region where axons are excited only by the C pulse is farther from the electrode. Finally, local potential summation can occur in the farthest region if the local potentials produced by the C pulses are still sufficient to sum with the weak T pulses. The duration of local potential summation is shortened by higher-current C pulses, however. By comparing this condition to the equal-current pulses condition, then, the contribution of the SNP can be measured and the duration of local potential summation can be reduced.

These effects depend on the relative intensity of the C and T pulses, not on their absolute intensity. The addition and subtraction of RRP, SNP, and SubNP effects is greater when the ratio of intensities is greater.

ARPs are normally measured in single neurons by delivering a T pulse two times threshold. If the T pulses are twice the current of the C pulses in behavioral experiments, however, more axons are stimulated by the higher-current pulses, so that refractory period effects contribute a smaller portion of the variance. Higher ratios (large pulse/small pulse) are safer for eliminating RRP effects but reduce the signal-noise ratio (ARP firings/total firings). Ratios (large pulse/small pulse) of 1.4 or 1.5 are often used in behavioral experiments because they add and subtract most RRP, SNP, and SubNP effects without reducing the signal-to-noise ratio as much as double-current pulses. In all conditions, the lower-current pulses should be the same size as the equal-current pulses, so that the central refractory-period region is held constant.

To summarize, only ARPs contribute to the rise in E when higher-current T pulses are used. RRPs and SubNPs are added when equal-current pulses are used. SNPs are added when higher-current C pulses are used. Local potential summation is reduced when higher-current C pulses are used. The theoretical effects of stimulating a homogeneous bundle of axons with identical poststimulation excitability cycles are shown in Figure 6-6 (from Appendix I). Most importantly, if a population of axons with different ARPs is excited, the slope of the E curve defines the distribution of ARPs when higher-current T pulses are used.

Results using unequal-current C and T pulses

Data from self-stimulation (left) and stimulation-elicited circling (right) are shown in Figure 6-7. The E values have been normalized so that E values range from 0 to 1.0 in all three conditions. As compared with the equal-current condition, the higher-current C pulses reduced local potential summation at C-T intervals of 0.2 and 0.4 msec, and increased E at 2 to 5 msec. The higher-current T pulses reduced E slightly at 1.2 msec in the self-stimulation data, and at 1.2 and 2.0 msec in the circling data.

These data suggest that ARPs account for the sharp rise from 0.4 to 1.2 msec in the self-stimulation data. RRP effects are small (Bielajew et al., 1982). In the more reliable circling data, RRPs account for 5–10 percent at C-T intervals of 1.2 and 2.0 msec. SNP contributions are large (10 to 40 percent) at longer C-T intervals in both experiments. Local potential summation was reduced at 0.2 and 0.4 msec using a larger C pulse. This is convenient because it reduces the overlap between the local potential summation and ARPs (Mili-

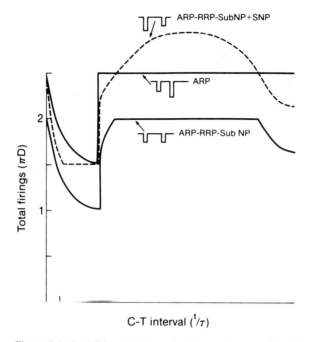

Figure 6-6. Total firings due to equal and unequal current C and T pulses. Based on the model of Figure 6-5, the total number of firings in an ideal axon bundle are calculated at each C-T interval. All axons are assumed to have the same threshold and ARP. When higher-current T pulses are used, the excitability curve is a step function at the ARP. The total firings are measured in units of the area of the circle of excitation at rest in Figure 6-5; that is, π times the diameter *(D)*.

aressis, 1981). There is no evidence of a depression interval. The refractory period hypothesis, therefore, accounts for all of these complex relationships.

Subnormal periods

There is a second important reason for using higher-current T pulses to measure the refractory period curve: in some cases, E values exceed 1.0 due to contributions of the SubNP. The SubNP can only be observed using longer C-T intervals. Self-stimulation data using C-T intervals up to 100 msec are shown in Figure 6-8. A 50 percent decline in E was observed at C-T intervals from 10 to 100 msec.

The evidence that this is due to the SubNP is seen in the second panel: Higher-current T pulses erased the decline in E. The explanation for why E values were above 1.0 at C-T intervals of 5.0 and 10.0 msec is that the SubNP lasted longer than the C-C interval and so E was better before the onset of the SubNP than during the single-pulse condition used for comparison. When the SubNP was erased, the high points at 5 and 10 msec dropped to $E = 1.0$. The

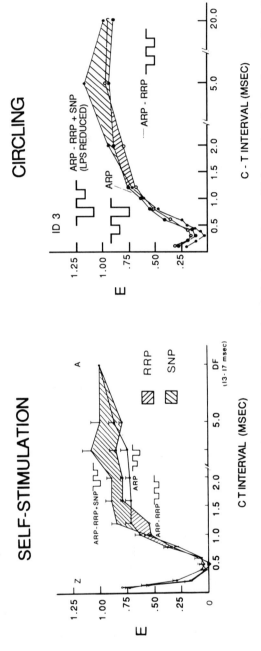

Figure 6-7. Behavioral measurement of ARPs, RRPs and SNPs. Left: Paired-pulse effectiveness (*E*) for equal- and unequal-current C and T pulses for MFB self-stimulation (after Yeomans, 1979). Right: The same for circling evoked from midbrain stimulation (after Yeomans & Linney, 1985). In both cases, the data in unequal-current conditions were normalized so that *E* ranged from 0 to 1.0. The effects attributable to RRP and SNP are shown in slashed regions.

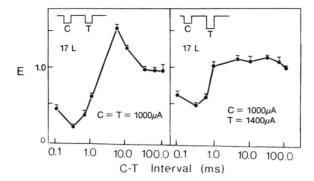

Figure 6-8. Behavioral measurement of subnormal periods for MFB self-stimulation. The decline from 5 to 100 msec is attributable to the subnormal period, since this decline was not seen when larger-current T pulses were delivered. C-T interval is plotted on a log scale.

end of the SubNP cannot be seen and must be longer than 100 msec. In addition, larger RRP effects were also observed at the C-T interval of 1.0 msec and erased by the larger-current T pulses.

This SubNP effect is only seen in occasional electrode placements. The occurrence of large RRP and SubNP effects may be related to the recruitment of high-threshold axons at high currents. To observe long C-T intervals, high currents and long C-C intervals must be used.

Because SubNPs can be large and the SubNP can reduce the effectiveness of the single-pulse conditions, estimates of refractoriness should be based on the rise in E from 0.3 to 5 or 10 msec (with local potential summation removed) rather than the absolute E value (Yeomans et al., 1985). The absolute E value is altered when the following C pulse is presented in the SubNP.

Distribution of absolute refractory periods

The gradual rise in E from 0.4 to 1.2 msec suggests that the directly excited MFB neurons mediating self-stimulation have a range of ARPs. Since ARPs are relatively fixed for individual neurons, the slope of the E curve measures the behavioral effect of neurons of a given ARP at each C-T interval. The distribution of ARPs, weighted by their behavioral effect, can be estimated from the slope of the rising E curve for higher current T pulses.

In behavioral studies, the neurons are weighted by their effect on the stimulation-evoked behavior. When recording from units one can never be sure whether these units have any behavioral significance. The property of weighting the behavioral importance of neurons of different types is a great strength of the behavioral method that is found with no other method. A second advantage is that this method measures the properties of large populations of stimulated axons.

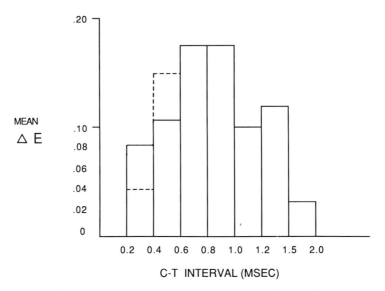

Figure 6-9. Refractory periods of axons mediating MFB self-stimulation. E values were taken from several studies in which local potential summation was below .25 at 0.2 msec. The mean E at a C-T interval of 0.4 msec was .07, at 0.6 msec was .17, at 0.8, was .34, and so on. The differences in mean E are shown to estimate the distribution of refractory periods. The dotted lines at 0.2 to 0.4 and 0.4 to 0.6 show the distribution if half of the contribution at 0.4 msec is attributed to residual local potential summation.

Only a few curves have been obtained using higher-current T pulses and these differ only slightly from curves using equal-current pulses at currents below 650 μA. Equal-current pulses, then, were used to estimate the distribution of ARPs in Figure 6-9. The estimate is based on 24 electrodes using 250 μm electrode tips at currents from 110 to 630 μA at frequencies from 25 to 110 Hz. Electrodes with E greater than 0.20 at a C-T interval of 0.4 msec were excluded to minimize local potential summation contamination. The dotted lines show the estimate if half of the effect at 0.4 msec is due to local potential summation rather than refractory periods. Refractory periods are spread evenly from 0.4 to 1.5 msec, with the heaviest contribution from 0.6 to 1.0 msec. This range is consistent with the range of ARPs observed from MFB units.

Gratton and Wise (1985) have done a finer-grained analysis, and measured the slope of the E curve (Figure 6-10). The rises in their refractory period curves are especially sharp from 0.5 to 0.6 msec, and from 0.7 to 0.8 msec. The "bumps" on the refractory period curve occur at the same intervals repeatedly. The first bump at 0.5 msec was blocked with peripheral injections of the muscarinic blocker, atropine.

Spatial variables that alter refractory period estimates

In Chapter 3, four spatial variables were found to alter the number of neurons recruited: current, tip size, substrate location relative to the tip, and thresholds

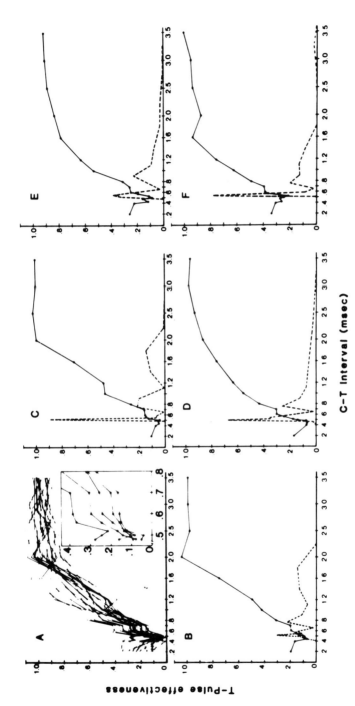

Figure 6-10. Gratton and Wise's (1985a) data for MFB self-stimulation for six electrodes. Solid lines: mean E values; dotted lines: differences in mean E. For panel A, each replication for a single electrode is shown, so that the reliability of the plateau from 0.6 to 0.7 can be seen.

of the axons. These spatial variables also alter the distribution of refractory periods. That is, since low-threshold neurons tend to have shorter refractory periods, altering spatial variables can alter the refractory period distribution.

Increasing the tip size has two effects: (1) the tip displaces axons in the center of the ARP region (Figures 6-11A and 6-5); (2) the current density at the tip is reduced so that high-threshold axons are harder to excite. Lowering the current reduces the number of axons excited, especially high-threshold axons.

Figure 6-11B shows refractory period curves for very large (0.6 mm^2 tip surface area) and very small (.01 mm^2) tips at various currents using equal-current C and T pulses. The refractory period curves shift to slightly longer C-T intervals using smaller tips or higher currents. This suggests that high-threshold axons with longer refractory periods can also contribute to MFB self-stimulation. When larger tips and lower currents are used, only the shorter refractory period axons are recruited. As discussed in Chapter 4, these high-threshold axons have the properties of the unmyelinated axons of midbrain dopamine cells.

In theory, different electrode placements can also alter the population of stimulated axons. If the electrode tip is outside of the bundle, high-threshold axons are harder to recruit. The refractory period distribution is altered if the electrode excites competing or inhibitory axons with different refractory periods. Refractory period curves represent the net excitatory effects at each C-T interval rather than only the pure excitatory effects.

Spatial variables have even greater effects on RRP, SNP, and local potential summation contributions. These are obtained in fringe regions (Figure 6-5) so that their contributions depend on how many neurons are found in the fringe regions relative to the above-threshold region. For example, if large tips are used, the center of the field, where ARP effects occur, is removed. In this case, local potential summation can be higher (Figure 6-11, top). Local potential summation can be reduced by using small tips, by increasing the current, or by placing the electrodes accurately in the bundle, thereby reducing the fringe relative to the center. These procedures in theory have a similar effect on RRP, SNP, and SubNP effects.

Therefore, the regions drawn in Figures 6-5 and 6-6 do not account for the location of the axon bundle. The number of axons recruited in each region also depends on how many axons are located in that region.

CONDUCTION FACTORS

Following axonal stimulation, action potentials must conduct to synapses to become behaviorally effective. If conduction is via fine axon terminals or collaterals, action potentials initiated by T pulses in the RRP may fail to conduct through the finer branches at short C-T intervals.

When stimulating axons at a long distance from the terminals, however, the speed of conduction can alter the time that the action potentials arrive at the fine terminals. Action potentials initiated during the RRP conduct more slowly

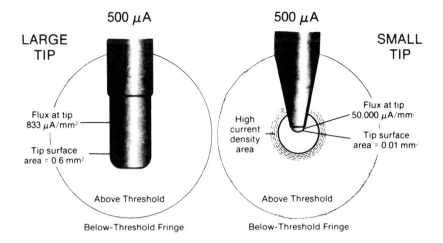

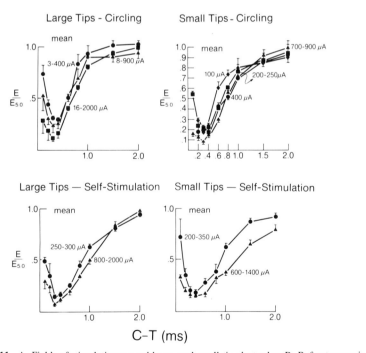

Figure 6-11. A. Fields of stimulation around large- and small-tip electrodes. B. Refractory periods curves shift to the right when higher currents or larger tips are used. Upper panels, refractory period data for circling evoked by midbrain stimulation, large tips on the left, small tips on the right. Lower panels, refractory period data for MFB self-stimulation, large tips on the left, small tips on the right. E values are divided by the E at a C-T interval of 5.0 msec, so that SubNP effects do not contaminate these measures of the refractory periods (Yeomans et al., 1985).

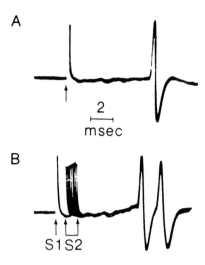

Figure 6-12. Conduction of action potentials during the RRP and SNP (Kocsis et al., 1979). Antidromic spikes were evoked by callosal stimulation 15 mm from a visual cortex recording electrode. A. Conduction of a single action potential at a latency of 7.7 msec following the stimulus artefact shown by the arrow. B. Paired pulses delivered at C-T intervals from 0.9 to 2.0 msec. The C pulse (S1) triggered the oscilloscope at the same time for all sweeps. The different T pulse artifacts (S2) are shown at different C-T intervals. Despite the variation in stimulus latency, however, the second spike follows the first spike at an unvarying latency of about 1.7 msec.

than normal, and action potentials initiated during the SNP conduct more rapidly. Therefore, action potentials do not arrive at the terminals at the same interval as the C-T interval. In fact, if the conduction distance to the terminals is long enough, all paired firings initiated at C-T intervals less than a few milliseconds can arrive at the synapses at virtually the same interval (the end of the RRP) independent of the C-T interval of delivery at the axons (Kocsis et al., 1979) (Figure 6-12). In this case, downstream synapses cannot account for excitability changes at these intervals, since there is no difference in the interval of arrival of the action potentials at the synapses.

Determination of the length of axons from stimulation site to synapses (Chapter 7), then, is important in associating the rise in the paired-pulse curve with axonal, rather than synaptic, excitability changes. MFB self-stimulation axons appear to have strong SNPs at 5 msec (Yeomans, 1979) and conduct at least 3 mm beyond lateral hypothalamus (Shizgal et al., 1980). Midbrain circling sites have axons at least 5 mm long with similar SNPs (Yeomans & Linney, 1985;

Tehovnik & Yeomans, 1986). Downstream synapses, then, cannot modify the results for these systems at C-T intervals below 5 msec.

Synaptic factors might be important, however, when C-T intervals in the SubNP or longer are involved. SubNPs will slow the conduction of T pulse action potentials, thereby increasing the discriminability of C-T intervals for synapses.

SYNAPTIC FACTORS

Smith and Coons (1970) found that after the refractory period the current threshold for MFB self-stimulation increased as C-T interval increased from 5 to 200 msec. The size of the increase varied from 15 to 50 percent and correlated positively with the current used. This increase was attributed to a decline in temporal summation at long C-T intervals. This finding has been observed in less than half of the animals tested in other laboratories, however (Shizgal et al., 1980; Bielajew & Shizgal, 1982; Bielajew, personal communication). Figure 6-8, left, shows one example of this effect measured by the decrease in E rather than increase in current.

The increase in current threshold (or decrease in E) could also be due to the decline in excitability in axons in the SubNP. The SubNP has been found to last for hundreds of milliseconds and produce up to 40 percent decreases in excitability (Raymond & Lettvin, 1978; Swadlow & Waxman, 1978). If the SubNP is responsible for the change in behavioral data, higher current T pulses, which block SubNP contributions, should prevent the rise in threshold. Figure 6-8 shows that the decline in E (that is, the increase in frequency threshold) at long C-T intervals is eliminated using higher current T pulses. Therefore, the Smith and Coons result is attributable to the SubNP, and cannot be accounted for by temporal summation. To conclude, synaptic contributions to the E curve for MFB self-stimulation appear to be slight.

CONCLUSIONS

Refractory period effects can be quantitatively measured by the trade-off between frequency and C-T interval, comparing the required frequency in paired-pulse conditions to the required frequency in single-pulse conditions. The decline in T-pulse effectiveness *(E)* at C-T intervals below 0.3 msec is due to a decline in local potential summation in neurons not quite excited by C pulses. The subsequent rise in E is due to recovery from refractoriness in neurons that were excited by the C pulses. The effects of local potential summation can be separated from refractory periods by using anodal C pulses followed by cathodal T pulses, or by C pulses of higher cathodal current than T pulses.

By delivering higher-current T pulses, the poststimulation excitability curve is simplified to a step function for each axon, with the step at the end of the ARP of each axon. When a population of axons is stimulated, the slope of the

E curve measures the distribution of ARPs of the directly excited neurons producing the response. The refractory period distribution varies widely from site to site and from behavior to behavior. The refractory period distribution in a single site can be altered by spatial variables (such as current, pulse duration, tip surface area, and distance from the tip) that alter the recruitment of long- and short-refractory-period axons. The contributions of RRPs, SNPs, and SubNPs can be separately measured by the use of unequal-current C and T pulses. Synaptic contributions to E appear to be slight for MFB self-stimulation.

HISTORICAL NOTE

Paired-pulse experiments were central to neurophysiology from its inception. Refractory periods were discovered by stimulating peripheral motor nerves containing hundreds of axons and observing muscle contractions (Helmholtz, 1854; Gotch & Burch, 1899). Larger muscle twitches resulted when the C-T interval was larger than the refractory period. This nerve-muscle preparation was also used in the discovery of conduction velocities (Helmholtz, 1850), collision (Lucas, 1917), SNP, SubNP (Lucas, 1971a; Erlanger & Gasser, 1937) synaptic delay, and summation phenomena (Sherrington, 1906).

Paired-pulse experiments, however, have had reduced importance in biophysical neurophysiology since the 1930s. The poststimulation excitability function cannot be easily described mathematically, which has been a problem in an increasingly mathematical field (Jack et al., 1983). Single axons are more often characterized by time constant and length constant, the two passive electrical properties of cells which determine local potential and conduction velocity parameters, respectively. In units, the exponential equations for these constants are easy to handle mathematically.

In brain stimulation, however, many units are excited and their effects integrated into a response. It is, therefore, harder to determine the properties of the many different underlying units. Higher-current T pulses reduce the poststimulation excitability curve to a step function at the ARP. This step function allows characterization of neural populations when many neurons are involved. This makes paired-pulse stimulation much more useful in brain stimulation than in single-neuron studies.

This chapter has been long and technical. There had to be theory to explain the effects of unmatched C and T pulses. There had to be empirical evidence and tests of the model. The beauty of paired-pulse stimulation is that axon excitation has been well studied, so that complex quantitative models can be derived and tested. The world of electrical stimulation of nerve has been inhabited by many great scientists—Helmholtz, Lucas, Sherrington, Gasser, Katz, and Hodgkin, to name a few. The ideas are rich and elegant. Perhaps brain stimulators can stand on the shoulders of these giants to provide a similar richness and elegance to our field.

FURTHER READINGS

Erlanger, J., & Gasser, H.S. *Electrical Signs of Nervous Activity*. London: Oxford University Press, 1937. Especially valuable for paired-pulse stimulation review.

Waxman, S. (ed.). *Physiology and Pathobiology of Axons*. New York: Raven Press, 1978. Several good chapters on excitability and conduction properties of axons.

7

Two-electrode Stimulation
of Axon Bundles

The most powerful methods for mapping the anatomy of behavior-producing axonal systems use two electrodes concurrently. In this chapter, two double-pulse studies are discussed where C pulses are delivered via one electrode and T pulses are delivered via a second electrode. By placing two electrodes lateral to one another across a bundle of axons, the current–distance relationship can be estimated by the refractoriness observed when the two fields of stimulation overlap. By placing two electrodes at different distances from one another along a bundle of axons, the length, trajectory, and conduction velocities of the axons can be estimated. Later, simultaneous stimulation through two electrodes is discussed, with reference to determining the direction of conduction along a bundle.

STIMULATION METHODS

When double-pulse stimulation is delivered via two electrodes, it is important to disconnect the unstimulated electrode from ground during the stimulating pulses (Figure 7-1). If current can flow between the cathode and the grounded second electrode, anodal excitation can occur via this second electrode (Figure 7-1, right). When double pulses are used, this anodal excitation can result in double stimulation of both sites. This anodal current can also alter the size and shape of the field of stimulation (Chapter 2).

In two-electrode studies, the effects of stimulating each electrode separately must also be tested. For example, for a two-electrode double-pulse experiment, the control conditions are double-pulse tests via each electrode separately. In addition, the two electrodes must often be matched with preliminary screening tests. Consequently, two-electrode experiments require more than twice the work of comparable one-electrode experiments.

BEHAVIORAL MEASUREMENT OF CURRENT–DISTANCE RELATIONSHIPS

The current–distance relationships of the behavior-relevant substrates determine the spatial resolution and selectivity of the stimulation. The current–distance

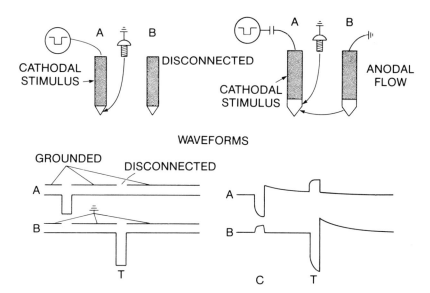

Figure 7-1. When two electrodes are used, electrode B must be disconnected when electrode A is delivering current, so that anodal current does not stimulate neurons near electrode B. Left, current correctly flows only from the skull screw to the cathodal electrode A and not from the disconnected electrode B. Right, current improperly flows from both the grounded electrode B and the skull screw.

data of Chapter 3, however, give only rough guidelines, since K estimates of units vary from about 50 to 10,000 μA/mm^2. In this section, the distribution of current–distance relationships is estimated for the axons mediating midbrain circling and MFB self-stimulation.

Fouriezos and Wise (1984) proposed a novel method for estimating the current–distance relationship. If two electrodes are placed side by side in a bundle, the fields of excitation overlap at higher currents, but not at low currents (Figure 7-2). The overlap in the fields can be measured by the refractoriness observed when stimulating concurrently through both electrodes. If C pulses are presented via one electrode, and T pulses via the second electrode, then behaviorally measured refractoriness is observed at short C-T intervals when the two fields overlap.

Refractoriness

Electrode pairs were placed in midbrain sites where circling is evoked (Yeomans et al., 1986b). Refractoriness was measured for each single electrode as in Chapter 6, then compared to refractoriness measured when C pulses were presented via one electrode and T pulses via the second electrode, or vice versa. When using two electrodes, $E = \{FT_{ct}/[(FT_{spa} + FT_{spb})/2]\} - 1$, where FT_{spa} is the required frequency when delivering single pulses via electrode a, and FT_{spb} is the required frequency when delivering single pulses via electrode b. Double-electrode refractoriness was defined as the difference between E at long

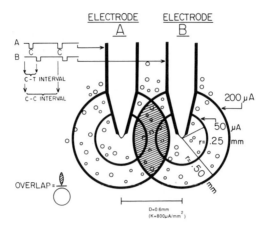

Figure 7-2. Fouriezos' method for behaviorally measuring the current–distance relationship. Two electrodes are placed across a bundle of axons. C pulses are delivered through electrode A and T pulses through electrode B. If the current is sufficient, axons in the region of overlap (cross-slashed area) will not be excited by the T pulses during their refractory period. Therefore, the radius of the fields of excitation can be estimated by the percent refractoriness at short C-T intervals, when the distance between electrodes is known (from Yeomans et al., 1986).

C-T intervals (2 and 5 msec) and short C-T intervals (0.2 and 0.4 msec) (Figure 7-3, left). Single-electrode refractoriness was defined as E at long C-T intervals (2 and 5 msec). Overlap was measured by the double-electrode refractoriness divided by the single-electrode refractoriness.

Double-electrode refractoriness is shown for two pairs in Figure 7-3. Refractoriness increased systematically as current increased. This is consistent with the idea that refractoriness is a measure of the overlap in the two stimulating fields. Furthermore, as interelectrode distance decreased, the level of refractoriness increased systematically.

Spatial summation

Spatial summation also increased systematically with overlap (Figure 7-3). Summation is measured by E at C-T intervals of 2.0 and 5.0 msec. Summation increased from .58 to .87 as interelectrode distance decreased from .82 to .38 mm ($r = -.95$). There was a smaller increase in summation as current increased. This suggests that spatially distributed action potentials are less effective than action potentials arriving from a spatially compact locus. This large change in summation with interelectrode distance violates the assumption of the counter model, which states that all action potentials count equally.

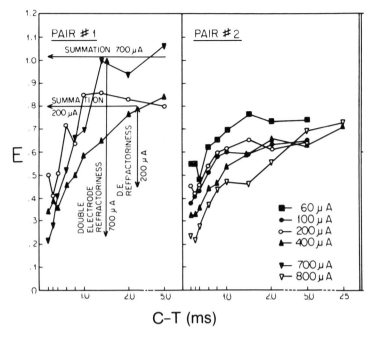

C-T (ms)

Figure 7-3. Refractoriness observed in the two-electrode experiment of Figure 7-2. In both cases the double-electrode refractoriness increased as the current of stimulation increased. The electrodes of pair #1 were closer together than pair #2, so the refractoriness observed was greater. In pair #1, the summation between electrodes also increased with current (Yeomans et al., 1986).

Model of overlap

The model in Figure 7-2 shows the overlapping fields at different currents (Yeomans et al., 1986). The fields are shown as circles using the "ideal bundle" assumptions discussed in Chapter 3: (1) an infinite field of uniform density axons, (2) point source stimulation, (3) isotropic impedance, (4) the radius of the field of stimulation is defined by $I = Kr^2$, (5) all axons have the same current–distance constant, K. The area of intersection between the two circles, then, can be calculated at any interelectrode distance (D) and current (I). In Figure 7-2, $D = 0.6$ mm, $K = 800$ $\mu A/mm^2$, $I = 200$ μA, and so overlap $= .24$. The *overlap* is the area of intersection divided by the area of one circle.

Predictions of model

On Figure 7-4A, the overlap predicted by the model of Figure 7-2 is shown as a function of current. The predicted overlap is shown by the smooth light lines. The current has been divided by the interelectrode distance squared so that the predictions of overlap for different K values can be shown on one graph for different interelectrode distances.

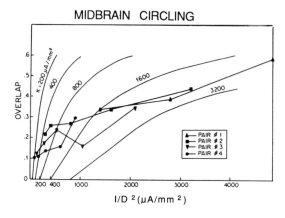

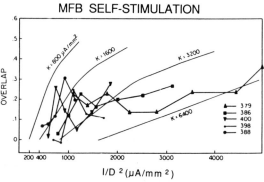

Figure 7-4. Increase in percent refractoriness ("overlap") with current in the two-electrode experiment. Current is divided by the square of interelectrode distance on the abcissa to correct for the different distances between electrodes. Above, circling from midbrain sites (Yeomans et al., 1986). Below, MFB self-stimulation (Fouriezos & Wise, 1984). Light lines show the predicted results if all axons have a single K value (Yeomans et al., 1986).

The data points represent the observed overlap taken from Figure 7-3 and two other electrode pairs. K was estimated for each data point by the location of the data point relative to the predicted K curves. At low values of I/D^2, K estimates were near 200 μA/mm^2. At high values of I/D^2, K estimates were near 3,000 μA/mm^2. This suggests that low threshold axons were excited at low current densities, and higher threshold axons were excited at higher current densities. To achieve an average of 3,000 μA/mm^2 at the highest currents, axons with thresholds above 4,000 μA/mm^2 on average must have been added to the lower threshold axons recruited at lower currents. Each current tested gives a new estimate of the K values of the axons added by the new current. A distribution of K values can be generated in this way.

Fouriezos and Wise's self-stimulation data are shown on Figure 7-4B. The distribution of K was found to be similarly wide—that is, from 1,000 to 8,000 μA/mm^2. The data were more variable for self-stimulation than for circling, however. The thresholds for self-stimulation axons were generally higher than circling axons. This is consistent with the longer refractory periods and slower conduction velocities of self-stimulation axons. Since MFB axons of midbrain dopamine cells have K values that range from 3,600 to 8,000 μA/mm^2, dopamine axons can be recruited only at the higher currents (Yeomans et al., 1986a).

Several criticisms of the model and results can be made. First, exceedingly reliable data (errors less than 5 percent) are required to obtain threshold distributions, so this method is not practical in most systems.

Second, at high currents the field of stimulation extended beyond the limits of the behaviorally effective bundle, so the assumption of an infinite bundle leads to an error in this case. The obtained overlap, however, should rise sharper than the predicted curves, since the overlap is greatest between the electrodes, not on the edges of the bundle. This factor, then, cannot account for the slower rise than predicted.

Fields of excitation

Another criticism is that refractoriness measures are contaminated by RRP, SNP, and SubNP contributions in the double-electrode experiment. Using two electrodes, the relative intensity of C and T pulses cannot be controlled for each axon as they can in the single-electrode experiment. The recovery for each axon, then, cannot be reduced to a step function.

The fields of excitation for double electrodes assuming a single K are shown more accurately in Figure 7-5. The C pulse is delivered via the left electrode and the T pulse via the right electrode. The solid lines show the predictions of the model of Figure 7-2, where two firings are found only in the region of overlap. In the region of overlap nearest the right electrode, the current density is high for both pulses and so recovery occurs at the ARPs of the axons. Farther from the right electrode, RRP and SNP effects occur. The distance from the electrode delivering the T pulse is critical, since the recovery is independent of the C pulse intensity when that pulse is above threshold. Outside of the overlap region, double firings are added by the SNP. Note that the RRP, SNP, and SubNP regions are smaller than in the single-electrode experiment (Figure 6-7), due to the partial overlap, but larger relative to the region of overlap, due to shrinkage of the ARP region (see Appendix I).

The problem for the current–distance model is that the SNP region makes the double-firing region larger than the overlap region of Figure 7-2. Therefore, double-electrode refractoriness will be slightly higher and occur at longer C-T intervals than predicted by that model.

The region of local potential summation is complicated since it depends on both C and T pulse intensity. That is, it is not determined by the radius from one electrode, but by the summation of currents from the two radii. At a C-T interval of 0, the region of local potential summation (LPS$_0$) is an oval, in particular, one of the ovals of Cassini (Appendix I). At a C-T interval of τ, the

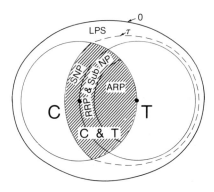

Figure 7-5. Fields of excitation in the two-electrode experiment. In this case, the radius of the field of excitation is equal to the interelectrode distance. Two firings can occur in the cross-slashed area, when C-T intervals are longer than the ARP near the T electrode. T pulse firings are added during the RRP or lost during the SubNP in the next region, and added or lost during the SNP in the region beyond the C electrode. The size of the regions has been drawn for excitability cycle A of Figure 6-1. Single firings occur following the C or T pulse independent of C-T interval in the regions marked with a C or T. A single firing can occur in the LPS fringe region at very short C-T intervals. The outer oval shows the region when the C-T interval is 0; the dashed line shows the region when the C-T interval is τ, the time constant of the axons.

local potential summation region (LPSτ) is much smaller than in the one-electrode experiment. Also, the LPS region is smaller nearer the C electrode than the T electrode, since local potential summation is reduced by higher-current C pulses.

The fields of excitation are shown for the case where the radius of C-pulse excitation equals the interelectrode distance. When the overlap is less, RRPs, SNPs, and SubNPs contribute a larger percentage to double-electrode refractoriness than ARPs. The size of these regions changes as the C-T interval changes, of course. When the thresholds of the axons vary, the boundaries are less focused also. The fields are shown quantitatively for several interelectrode distances in Appendix I.

Single-electrode refractory period tests can never be a perfect control for double-electrode refractoriness. If C and T pulses are equal in current, SNP contributions do not exist and RRP and SNP contributions give a smaller percentage to the observed refractoriness. For this reason, higher-current C pulses, which include the SNP, may be a better control, although the size of the regions is still not perfectly matched.

Conclusions

The K estimates obtained in the two-electrode experiment fall in the range estimated for units, and suggest that a wide range of thresholds are found in the midbrain axons mediating circling. This range of thresholds is consistent with the wide range of refractory periods and conduction velocities observed for these axons in other experiments. The K estimates for MFB self-stimulation are wide also, but much higher on average, which is consistent with the longer refractory periods and slower conduction velocities found for those axons than for axons mediating circling. Several sources of error for these K estimates are discussed.

THE COLLISION EXPERIMENT

The collision experiment determines whether two stimulating electrodes are both exciting the same axon. By moving the stimulating electrodes and testing for collision, the path taken by this axon can be determined. At the same time, the collision method estimates the conduction velocity of the axon.

Excitation of an axon evokes two action potentials, one traveling in the normal (orthodromic) direction toward the terminals, and a second traveling back toward the cell body (antidromic). If an axon is excited simultaneously at two sites along its length, then four action potentials are evoked. The two action potentials traveling toward one another collide and erase one another (Figure 4-4, top). Therefore, only one action potential is recorded from either end of the axon when collision occurs.

If one site is stimulated with a C pulse and the second site stimulated later with a T pulse, collision does not occur when the C-T interval is long enough for the first action potential to pass beyond the second electrode. Consequently, two action potentials reach the terminals per pulse pair instead of one. This is the same as the refractory period experiment, in that one or two action potentials reach the terminals per pulse pair, as a function of C-T interval. Collision does not depend on whether the C pulse is presented via the distal or proximal electrode—that is, the result is symmetrical.

The period during which collision occurs (the *collision interval*) is usually roughly equal to the ARP plus the conduction time. Conduction velocity, then, can be estimated by dividing conduction distance by the collision interval minus the ARP. This estimate is not always perfect, however. For example, when recording from cell bodies, the recorded collision interval can be different from the sum of the conduction time and the ARP (Fuller & Schlag, 1976).

The collision experiment is also similar to the current–distance experiment. When collision occurs, half of the action potentials are removed. The recovery from collision occurs very rapidly at relatively short C-T intervals. The two main differences result from the fact that the second electrode is down rather than across the axon. First, the conduction time between electrodes is added to the refractory period, and, second, local potential summation is not evident.

If synapses occur between the two electrodes, this simple collision result cannot occur. First, potentials cannot conduct antidromically across most synapses. Second, presynaptic action potentials do not always produce postsynaptic action potentials, and if they do, the outputs are delayed and unreliable. Therefore, "transynaptic collision" will be less reliable, and will depend on whether C pulses are presented via the presynaptic or postsynaptic electrode. Therefore, transynaptic collision, if it occurs at all, is weak and asymmetric (Chapter 8).

Consequently, the criteria for axonal collision are (1) that one of the two action potentials is removed whenever the C-T interval is shorter than a relatively fixed interval, (2) that this collision interval is longer than the ARP of either stimulation site, by an amount consistent with the conduction time between sites, and (3) that the collision interval is the same when the C pulses are delivered to either electrode—that is, it shows symmetry. Evidence of collision of this sort suggests that two stimulating sites are connected by continuous axons (Lipski, 1981; Schlag, 1978).

Conduction velocity

Conduction velocity is closely correlated with fiber diameter (Figure 7-6). In large myelinated fibers, the relationship $CV/D = 6$, where CV is conduction velocity in msec and D is outside fiber diameter in μm, is a good approximation (Hursch, 1939; BeMent, 1981). For unmyelinated fibers, the ratio is nearer 2, and for the smallest myelinated fibers the ratio is near 4 (Boyd, 1964; BeMent, 1981). There is usually an overlap in conduction velocities of small myelinated and large unmyelinated fibers (Paintal, 1978). Conduction velocity is also closely correlated with the distance between nodes of Ranvier, called the *internodal length*.

Collision-like effects in behavioral studies

Collision-like effects were measured in the nerve-muscle preparation by Lucas (1917b). The size of muscle twitches increased when the C-T interval exceeded the collision interval. Collision is not difficult to obtain when stimulating peripheral nerves, because the electrodes can be attached to the isolated nerve, and very high currents can be used without danger of activating other nervous tissue.

In brain tissue, it is difficult to align the electrodes in the same place in a bundle, and the currents must be limited. Collision, therefore, occurs in only part of the stimulated axons when the alignment is imperfect (Figure 7-7). Also, some axons may not be parallel with the others in the bundle, or may terminate before the second electrode.

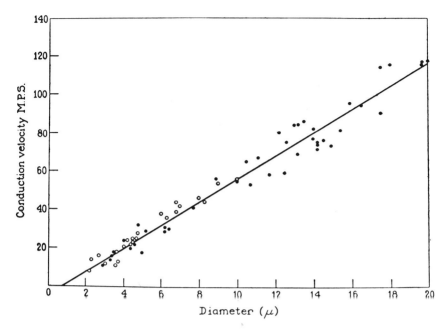

Figure 7-6. Conduction velocity increases with axon diameter in a nearly linear fashion for large peripheral nerve axons (Ruch et al., 1965, after Hursch, 1939).

Figure 7-7. Collision depends on electrode alignment. If the electrodes are misaligned, then the percent collision is likely to increase as the stimulating current is increased. Left, no collision due to low current (shown by small circles around electrodes) and no axons stimulated by both electrodes. Right, partial collision due to high current (shown by large dashed circles around electrodes) and several axons stimulated by both electrodes. This model is schematic (Shizgal et al., 1980).

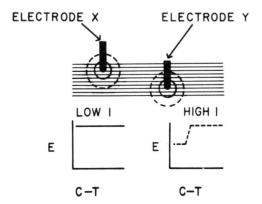

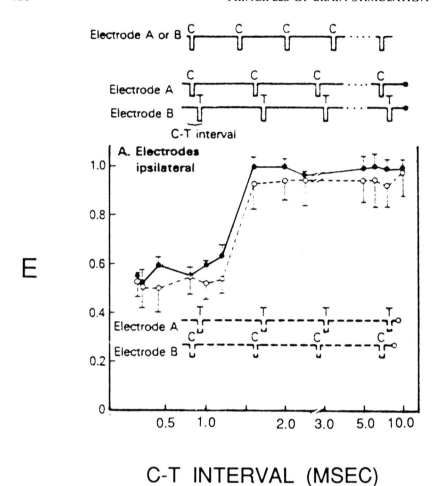

C-T INTERVAL (MSEC)

Figure 7-8. Behaviorally measured collision in MFB self-stimulation. Electrode A was placed in the lateral hypothalamus; electrode B was placed in the ventral tegmental area 3 mm caudally. C pulses were presented via electrode A and T pulses via electrode B, or vice versa. E was calculated by comparing the frequency threshold in paired-pulse experiments to the single-pulse conditions where T pulses are omitted for each electrode. The recovery occurred at C-T intervals between 1.2 and 1.6 msec, or much longer than the refractory period experiment. The percent collision was 50 percent in this experiment (Shizgal et al., 1980).

Shizgal et al. (1980) studied collision with two self-stimulation electrodes placed in the trajectory of the MFB. One electrode was placed in the lateral hypothalamus (LH), and the second electrode was placed about 3 mm caudally in the ventral tegmental area (VTA). The currents were adjusted so that the frequency required to produce bar-pressing at each of the two sites was the same. E was calculated as described above for current–distance estimates.

E values rose sharply at C-T intervals from 1.0 to 2.0 msec (Figure 7-8).

These critical C-T intervals were 0.4 to 1.0 msec longer than the single-electrode refractory periods (0.4 to 1.2 msec). In addition, these results differed from single-electrode paired-pulse curves in several ways:

1. No drop at C-T intervals from 0.1 to 0.4 msec was observed. Local potential summation cannot occur when the C and T pulses are delivered far apart spatially.
2. E values never approached 0 at the shortest C-T intervals. Collision cannot occur in all axons unless the electrodes are perfectly aligned with the bundle and all the axons maintain the same trajectory relative to the electrodes.
3. The results were the same whether C pulses were presented via the LH electrode or the VTA electrode—that is, symmetry was observed.
4. When the two LH electrodes were on opposite sides of the brain, no collision-like change in E was observed.

These results, then, satisfy the criteria for axonal collision described above.

These collision-like effects suggest that the MFB axons mediating self-stimulation can be excited by both LH and VTA electrodes. The axons must therefore be longitudinal fibers at least 3 mm in length, since that was the interelectrode distance. Since the collision intervals were 0.4- to 1.0-msec longer than the refractory periods, the conduction velocities must be roughly 3 to 8 m/second. Slower conduction velocities were observed in two caudal VTA placements (Bielajew & Shizgal, 1982). These conduction velocities suggest that fiber diameters are in the 0.7 to 2 μm range (Boyd, 1964).

These conduction velocities have been important in proving that dopamine-containing fibers, which have conduction velocities of 0.3 to 1.5 m/second (Guyenet & Aghajanian, 1978; German et al., 1980), cannot be the primary directly activated substrate for MFB self-stimulation (Gallistel et al., 1981; Yeomans, 1982; Chapter 4).

Collision maps describe the path of the behavior–producing axons

Similar collision effects have been observed in a variety of brainstem sites for circling (Yeomans & Linney, 1985; Tehovnik & Yeomans, 1986). The amount of collision varied with the alignment of the electrodes in the bundle. An electrode pair that was accurately aligned showed 0.4 to 0.6 collision at all currents tested. An electrode pair that was slightly misaligned showed an increase in collision from 0.3 to 0.7 as the current increased. This result is similar to the increase in double-electrode refractoriness in the current–distance experiment. From the variations in collision, Yeomans and Linney (1985) were able to estimate the optimal alignment of electrodes, and hence the path of the axons producing circling. In addition, spatial summation increased with current.

Figure 7-9 shows collision obtained between electrode pairs producing cir-

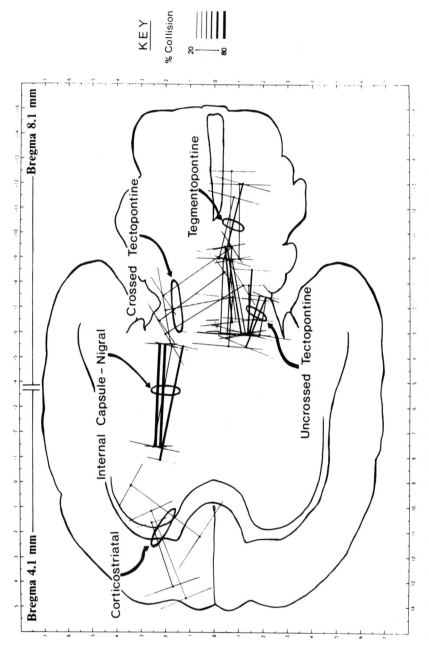

Figure 7-9. Behaviorally measured collision in sites where stimulation evokes circling. Where collision has been observed, sites are shown connected by a line. The percent collision is shown by the thickness of the line. The perpendicular line at each site shows the estimated radius of excitation, based on $K = 500 \ \mu\text{A/mm}^2$ (Yeomans & Tehovnik, 1988).

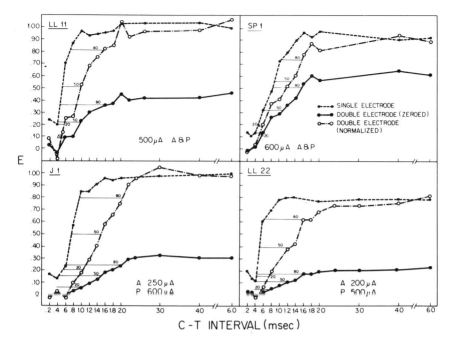

Figure 7-10. Conduction velocity estimates for circling evoked from midbrain and pons. The four panels show four electrode pairs, with one electrode in the pons and one in the midbrain. The dashed lines show refractory period curves (the mean of two electrodes). The collision data are shown in two ways. The solid line shows the collision curves lowered to a minimum E value of 0, so that the conduction times can be estimated by comparing the zeroed collision curves to the initial rise in the refractory period curves. The dotted line shows the same collision data normalized to range from E values of 0 to 1.00, so that the conduction times can be estimated by comparing the normalized collision curves to the whole refractory period curves.

cling. The thickness of each line shows the percent collision, so that the widest lines show the trajectories which best approximate the trajectory of the bundle of axons producing circling. The thin perpendicular lines are rough estimates of the field of excitation.

Conduction velocity distributions

For circling, the collision curves were not parallel to the refractory period curves, but diverged at higher E values (Figure 7-10). At low E values, the conduction times were near 0.1 msec, while at high E values the conduction times were near 0.8 msec. This divergence (which was not observed in the self-stimulation data) suggests that the curve is due fibers with a range of conduction velocities. The range of conduction velocities estimated (2–25 m/second) is consistent with conduction velocities (0.7–40 m/second) of tectobulbar axons (Yeomans & Linney, 1985; Miliaressis & Phillippe, 1983).

Technical problems in conduction velocity estimation

To obtain a conduction time estimate, the single-electrode curves must be compared with the double-electrode curves. These curves are different in several ways, however.

1. The two single-electrode curves are sometimes not identical.
2. The single-electrode curves include local potential summation, which often obscures the initial rise at E values below .20.
3. The collision curves include SNP contributions, while the single-electrode curves do not.
4. The single-electrode curves rise a total height of $E \sim 1.0$, while the double-electrode curves rise only partially, presumably due to imperfect alignment of the stimulation fields.

I will deal with each of these problems in order.

1. Differences in the two refractory period curves are rare, but can occur when one electrode stimulates the main axons, and the other electrode stimulates the initial segments, fine collaterals or axon terminals. Figure 7-11 shows a case where the two refractory period curves differed by a few tenths of a msec. The stimulating electrodes were in the motor cortex and in the medullary pyramid of rats, and the forelimb flexed when either electrode was stimulated. The refractory periods in cortex were much longer, probably because the pyramidal cells in cortex have low-threshold initial segments that are not myelinated.

The escape from collision occurs at the electrode where the T pulse is delivered, whether that electrode is proximal or distal from the cell. Therefore, the refractory period that must be subtracted from the collision interval is the refractory period at the electrode delivering the T pulse.

In Figure 7-11, the collision intervals for the C_{py}-T_{cx} collision curve were longer than the C_{cx}-T_{py} collision curve by about 0.4 msec, which suggests that asymmetrical collision might have occurred. When the refractory period for the electrode delivering the T pulse is subtracted, however, there is almost no difference between the conduction times for the two curves. There are two lessons here: (1) Use the refractory period for the T-pulse electrode to estimate conduction times; (2) Symmetry must be judged by conduction time data, and not collision interval data.

2. Local potential summation can be removed from the refractory period curves by using anodal C pulses or higher-current C pulses. Although anodal C pulses remove local potential summation completely they reduce the height of the refractory period curve severely at the same current (Appendix I). Local potential summation is best reduced by delivering C pulses that are higher in current then the T pulses. The proportion of the reduction increases with C-T interval (Miliaressis, 1981; Yeomans, 1979).

3. In the collision curves, recovery often occurs during the RRP or SNP, rather than at the end of the ARP (adding the conduction time to each of these). Figure 7-12 shows where these fields occur for the "ideal bundle." These

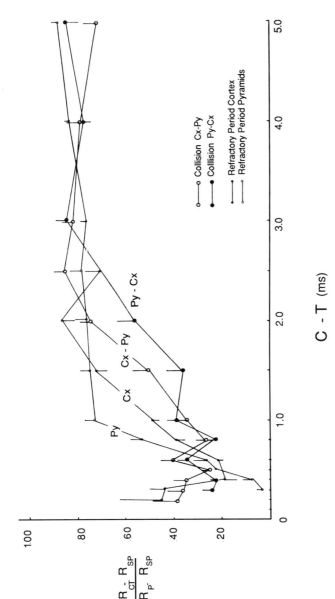

Figure 7-11. Refractory period and collision curves with electrodes in the motor cortex (Cx) and medullary pyramid (Py). The refractory period curves increased at C-T intervals from 0.4 to 1.0 msec in the pyramid, but at 0.6 to 2.0 msec in the cortex. The collision curves increased at C-T intervals from 0.8 to 2.5 msec when the C pulses were delivered to the cortex and the T pulses to the pyramid (Cx-Py), but from 0.8 (or 1.5) to 3.0 msec in the Py-Cx condition. These curves represent the average percent increase in forelimb flexion between single-pulse and peak responses from several rats.

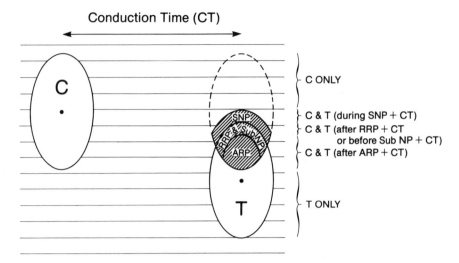

Figure 7-12. Model of fields of excitation in the collision experiment. The axons are assumed to be parallel and have identical thresholds and excitability cycles (Appendix I). C pulses are delivered to the center of the left field and T pulses to the center of the right field. The electrodes are misaligned in the bundle as in Figure 7-5. The number of firings conducted to the terminals in each axon is shown at the right. When two firings are conducted, the C-T interval must be appropriate, as shown at the right, that is, greater than the conduction time (CT) plus the ARP for axons passing through the region marked ARP, or equal to the conduction time plus the SNP for axons passing through the region marked SNP, or greater than the RRP plus the conduction time and less than the SubNP plus the conduction time for axons passing through the region marked RRP or SNP.

fields are very similar to those in the current–distance experiment (Figure 7-5) except that no local potential summation occurs and a conduction time is added. Therefore, at the highest E values collision curves rise more slowly than expected by the collision model of Figure 4-4. The percent contributions of RRP, SNP, and SubNP are discussed in Appendix I. The contaminating effects of RRPs, SNPs, and SubNPs can be reduced by increasing the size of the T pulses. Although this should improve the conduction velocity estimate at the top of the collision curves, the percent collision is harder to interpret than when the two electrodes are matched. Also, contaminating effects in the highest threshold axons or nonparallel axons cannot be removed reliably.

4. The problem with partial collision is that the axons producing collision tend to be lower-threshold axons with shorter refractory periods. The collision curve can be matched against the whole refractory period range, but the long refractory periods at the top of the curve reflect the activity of high-threshold axons that are less likely to produce collision.

One solution is to compare the collision curve with the lower part of the refractory period curve. That is, if 50 percent collision is observed, match the collision curve up against the first 50 percent of the refractory period curve. The problem with this method is that it goes too far—some longer refractory period axons will show collision as well, so this refractory period estimate is slightly too short. The method I have used is to take the mean of these two estimates in Figure 7-10 (Yeomans & Linney, 1985), but this is just a better approximation. This error becomes smaller as the percent collision increases.

In conclusion, conduction velocity estimates, like K estimates, are still an approximate science.

Downstream factors (axon terminal conduction, synaptic integration, subsequent refractory periods, etc.) are not a serious concern in conduction velocity estimates. These downstream factors are identical for the refractory period estimate and the collision interval estimate for the axons stimulated by both electrodes. Consequently, the differences between the refractory period and collision curves must be attributed to the conduction between the two electrodes rather than beyond the electrodes. Helmholtz (1850) and Lucas (1917b) used the same logic to prove that conduction velocity and refractory period estimates, respectively, could not be attributed to the speed of nerve-muscle synaptic transmission or of muscle activation.

Summary of collision

The length, path, and conduction velocities of behavior-producing axons are all measured in the collision experiment. The percent collision measures the proportion of the behavioral effects due to axons with different collision intervals. By finding which sites show collision, and which sites do not, rough path diagrams of functional systems can be drawn (e.g., Figure 7-9). Shizgal has likened this procedure to a "connect-the-dots" game, in which the stimulation sites are dots, and the collision tests show which dots are connected. When collision-like effects are not obtained, the two sites cannot be connected by behavior-producing axons.

Summation is a useful way to test the synaptic relatedness of sites. For example, summation between MFB and midbrain self-stimulation sites is usually between 40 and 70 percent (Bielajew et al., 1981; Kofman & Yeomans, 1988), which suggests that these sites feed into a common integrator. Summation between MFB and frontal cortex self-stimulation sites, however, is below 10 percent, which suggests that frontal cortex self-stimulation feeds through other reward systems (Schenk & Shizgal, 1982).

DIRECTION OF CONDUCTION

In behavioral systems, no simple method for determining the normal (orthodromic) direction of conduction is known. Traditional lesion methods for determining direction which involve separating the axons from their cell bodies or terminals can be helpful, but have many problems of their own. In most cases, therefore, the direction of conduction must be inferred from anatomical information alone. In most brain areas, however, pathways going in opposite directions are found near to one another.

Collision with spontaneous spikes

In units, direction can be determined by colliding antidromic spikes with spontaneous action potentials. A recording electrode is placed near a unit and the axon is stimulated with a separate electrode (Figure 7-13). If the recording is from the region of the cell body, the stimulus-evoked action potentials must have conducted back to the cell body in the antidromic direction. Spontaneous action potentials, which conduct only in the orthodromic direction, then, will collide with action potentials evoked at the same time by the stimulating electrode. Therefore, the stimulus-evoked action potential is erased whenever a spontaneous action potential is observed shortly before or after the stimulus. The spontaneous action potential must occur within one conduction time of the evoked action potential to erase it. When erasure of the evoked potential is observed, it is concluded that the recording electrode was observing antidromic evoked action potentials (Figure 7-13). This unit-recording method cannot determine the direction of the behavior-producing axons, however, since behavior cannot be recorded from the single neuron.

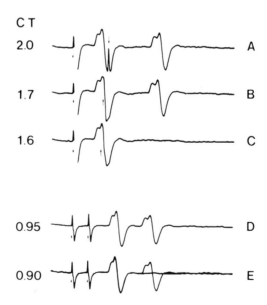

Figure 7-13. Collision and refractory period estimates in a unit driven by MFB stimulation (Rompre & Shizgal, 1986). The extracellular responses to stimulation with two pulses through a single electrode (traces D and E) or through separate electrodes (A-C) are shown. Two antidromic action potentials were observed when the stimulating pulses (arrows) were delivered through a single electrode at a C-T interval of 0.95 msec (Trace D). The second action potential occurred only half of the time at a C-T interval of .90 msec, due to the refractory period of the axon. When the two pulses were presented via separate electrodes, recovery occurred at a C-T interval of 1.7 msec, suggesting a conduction time of 0.8 ms. Calibration: 1mV, 1 msec.

Anode-cathode orientation

In axons, the conduction direction is influenced by the orientation of bipolar stimulating electrodes. The anode inhibits conduction (Rushton, 1949), so lower current thresholds for responses are obtained when the cathode is closer to the recording site than the anode. Consequently, thresholds for behavior should be lower when the cathode is closer to the terminals.

Szabo et al. (1972) tried this method in MFB self-stimulation. They found that less current was required when the rostral electrode of a bipolar pair served as cathode, in more cases than not. The problem with this method in behavioral systems, however, is that the rostral electrode may be placed closer to the relevant neurons, so that the lower threshold may reflect placement accuracy rather than electrode orientation. In behavioral systems, the contact between electrode and relevant neurons cannot be controlled accurately, and so differences in threshold are harder to interpret than with peripheral nerve stimulation.

Bielajew & Shizgal (1986) added several control procedures that clarify the interpretation. First, they studied electrode pairs that had already shown collision. To show collision, both electrodes must be accurately placed near the same behavior-producing axons.

Second, they reasoned that anodal inhibition cannot occur if the anodal stimulation is removed before the action potentials conduct to the anode. The conduction time was known from the collision experiment. They tested the block, then, at several pulse durations on the assumption that the anodal block would raise thresholds only at pulse durations longer than the conduction time. The strength-duration curve was measured using the LH electrode as anode and the VTA electrode as cathode, or vice versa (Figure 7-14). As control conditions, the two monopolar strength-duration curves were also tested.

In control conditions, thresholds in VTA generally were lower than in LH, although for electrode D-29 thresholds were equal. This is due to the higher concentration of MFB fibers in VTA. Next, thresholds were slightly lower for bipolar stimulation than for monopolar stimulation. This is probably due to the slight advantage of longitudinal over transverse stimulation (Chapter 3). This advantage is greater for the LH electrodes than the VTA electrodes, presumably due to the change in orientation of MFB fibers just rostral to VTA. These fibers turn dorsally as they enter the midbrain, and so are less longitudinal.

The strength-duration curves were found to be parallel to one another in all cases except when the LH was stimulated cathodally and the VTA anodally (LH − VTA +, on Figure 7-14). These curves fell more slowly at pulse durations longer than 0.5 msec; that is, at durations longer than the collision interval. Therefore, pulse durations longer than the collision interval were less effective when the anode was placed in the VTA, but not when the anode was placed in the LH. This suggests that the orthodromic direction is LH to VTA, with no evidence of VTA to LH conduction.

The size of the anodal block can be estimated by comparing the shift in the ratio of currents: I monopolar/I bipolar. For VTA cathodes (spots, right panels), this ratio was constant at all durations. For LH cathodes (circles, right panels),

STRENGTH - DURATION CURVE

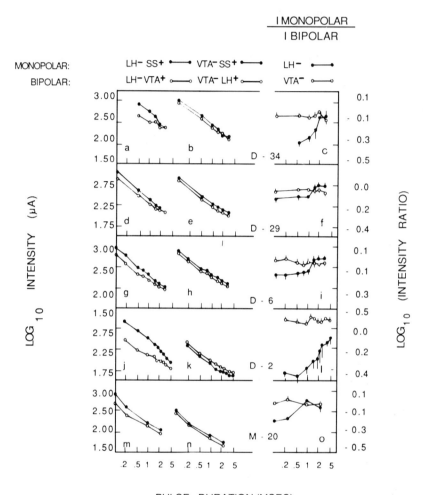

Figure 7-14. Directionality test for MFB self-stimulation (Bielajew & Shizgal, 1986). Strength-duration curves (shown on log-log coordinates) were taken as a baseline for each electrode (filled circles, left) in five different animals. When the return electrode was moved from the skull screw (SS+) to the second electrode, little change was observed for the VTA electrode (LH+), but an interaction was observed for the LH electrode (VTA+). The interaction is shown more clearly on the right where the current threshold in the monopolar condition is compared to the bipolar condition at each pulse duration.

this ratio changed sharply at durations longer than 0.5 msec. The 0.13 to 0.36 increase in the log ratio implies a 26 to 56 percent block by the VTA anode. The block did not correlate with the amount of collision, which ranged from 0.40 to 0.65, but correlated strongly with the currents used via the two electrodes. When the currents used for the two electrodes were perfectly matched

(D-29), the block was 26 percent; when the LH current was 4.3 times the VTA current (D-2), the block was 56 percent. Therefore, the block was stronger when the anodal blocking current was much greater than the cathodal threshold for a given site.

For the one pair of electrodes for which current thresholds were matched (D-29), anodal block was smaller than collision. This is consistent with the fact that anodal currents for block are higher than cathodal currents for stimulation (Chapter 3). Anodal block is much harder to observe via the higher-threshold electrode than the lower-threshold electrode. This problem makes the lack of a block via the LH electrode less conclusive when low currents were used via this electrode.

This direction test is painfully difficult, since it requires refractory period and collision testing followed by four different strength-duration curves. Also, the trajectory of the bundle to be stimulated must be considered. Finally, 5-msec anodal pulses can damage tissue, so platinum electrodes, or the lowest currents and shortest durations possible, must be used to prevent lesions.

In summary, there is still no simple way to determine conduction direction behaviorally when the anatomy allows for either direction. Bielajew and Shizgal's method is a big improvement theoretically, but requires collision testing and a minimum of four strength-duration curves. Finally, the amount of block is related to how well the current thresholds of the two electrodes are matched. This method needs to be tried in other systems than MFB self-stimulation to test its general validity.

FURTHER READINGS

Lipski, J. Antidromic activation of neurons as an analytic tool in the study of the central nervous system. *Journal of Neuroscience Methods,* 1981, *4,* 1–32.

Lucas, K. *Conduction of the Nerve Impulse* (E. Adrian, ed.). Aberdeen: University Press, 1917. This is a review of the first experiments using the collision method and measuring the supernormal period.

8

Future Directions in Cortical Stimulation, including Magnetic Stimulation and Transynaptic Collision

Electrical brain stimulation began with maps of the cerebral cortex. In this final chapter, some new approaches to cortical stimulation are evaluated, especially sight for the blind and transcranial electrical stimulation. Finally, the promising method of transynaptic collision is discussed.

VISUAL CORTEX STIMULATION OF BLIND HUMANS

Electrical stimulation of the human visual cortex has long been known to evoke pointlike sensations of light in a small part of the visual field (Foerster, 1926; Penfield & Jasper, 1954). Brindley and Lewin (1968) proposed that blind patients who have lost their sight by damage to the eye or optic pathway might have visual input restored by electrical stimulation of the intact visual cortex. An electrode array was surgically implanted against the surface of the visual cortex (in the longitudinal fissure of the occipital lobe) of one blind patient to test the feasability of this idea. Since then, a few more patients have been tested with arrays of up to 64 electrodes (Figure 8-1). The electrodes can be implanted permanently and activated nonintrusively either by connectors or by telemetry.

Electrical stimulation evokes pointlike visual sensations in the blind subjects that are essentially identical to those reported by normal patients undergoing brain surgery. The sensations are in most cases tiny white spots localized to a tiny part of the visual field. The spots appear to move with the eyes when voluntary eye movements occur, but remain fixed in space when reflexive eye movements are induced through the vestibular system (Brindley, 1982). These visual sensations are reliably evoked at a particular current (in the 0.8- to 5-mA range). Increases in current above threshold increase the brightness of the sensation. In a few sites, multiple spots have been reported.

The promise of this approach is that many sites might be stimulated together to produce visual patterns. These visual patterns could be arranged into letters

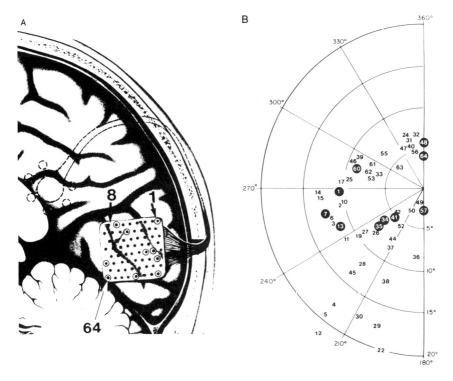

Figure 8-1. A. Placement of 64 platinum electrodes against the right medial occipital lobe of a blind human. The wires for each electrode pass out of the skull to a connector on the side of the head. The numbering of the electrodes from 1 to 64 is shown. B. The map of phosphene positions in the left visual field reported by the patient. The numbers refer to the electrode numbers (Evans et al., 1979).

or Braille dot patterns. Very complex patterns could be quickly delivered by computers. Alternatively, the electrodes might be activated by a television camera so that objects in front of the blind person could be detected.

In each subject, each site has been mapped in visual space. The subjects reliably report where the individual points are, in locations that correspond with the retinotopic map in most but not all sites. When combinations of several sites are stimulated, the subjects can describe the shape or letter made by these points. The subjects can be trained to use six-spot patterns to read Braille letters at rates as high as 30 letters per minute (Brindley & Rushton, 1974; Dobelle et al., 1976).

In spite of this remarkable success, the method has not been applied widely. First, the phosphenes interact when close together, perhaps due to the high currents required using surface electrodes. Therefore, only one letter has been presented at a time in the visual field. Also, at rates above 4 per second the signals tend to blur together. Therefore, reading rates are quite limited, and it is hard to see how these rates can improve substantially over Braille reading. Consequently, it is not yet certain whether the visual sensations evoked can help the blind to function better in any way that can justify the expense and danger of this surgical procedure (Brindley, 1982). Perhaps recent mappings of functional channels in visual cortex (Livingstone & Hubel, 1988) will allow better functional stimulation of visual cortex in humans.

TRANSCRANIAL STIMULATION OF HUMAN MOTOR CORTEX

Two new methods of stimulating the human cortex noninvasively have been developed in the last decade. Transcranial electrical stimulation is difficult because of the long distance from the scalp to the cortex and the high resistance of the skull and dura. Using high-voltage capacitor discharges (2,000 V, 0.1 μF capacitor, with a time constant of 10 msec), however, anodal electrical stimulation applied to the scalp over the motor cortex (Merton & Morton, 1980) can reliably evoke twitches of small muscles of the contralateral hand. Sensory structures (visual cortex or somatosensory cortex) can also be activated, but at much higher voltages.

A newer method is to apply magnetic fields to the brain by way of a ring-shaped, copper coil placed on the scalp (Figure 8-2). When a powerful current is applied to the coil, a strong magnetic field is created, which in turn induces a much smaller current through conductors inside the brain. Magnetic stimulation (0.9 to 2.1 Tesla) reliably evokes twitches in the same small muscles of the contralateral hand (Hess et al., 1987). One advantage of magnetic stimulation is that the stimulation does not produce the sharp, painful sensations in the scalp produced by electrical stimulation. A second advantage is that the EMG response to magnetic stimulation is slightly larger and shorter in duration than the response to electrical stimulation (Figure 8-4). The latency is slightly longer for magnetic stimulation (21–26 msec) than electrical stimulation (19–24 msec).

One practical value of transcranial stimulation is to test the functioning of the corticospinal tract in normal and brain-damaged patients. In peripheral nerve, conduction velocity has proved to be a sensitive measure of neural function (Dorfman et al., 1982). Many diseases, such as multiple sclerosis, involve central nervous conduction. Therefore, by comparing the latency of responses to cortical, cervical, and peripheral nerve stimulation, the conduction velocity of the corticospinal pathway (and possibly other pathways) can be accurately measured.

The motor map produced by transcranial stimulation is not nearly as detailed or as localized as the map observed by stimulating the cortex directly. Electrical stimulation works best roughly 3–4 cm from the midline over the motor cortex for the hand. Magnetic stimulation works better near the center of the head than directly over the motor cortex for the hand. When the inducing current in the coil is clockwise (looking down on the coil from above the head), the right hand is activated first; when the inducing current is counterclockwise, the left hand is activated first.

Recently, speech has been reported to be blocked by magnetic stimulation

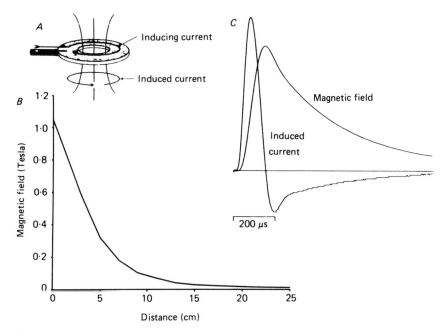

Figure 8-2. Magnetic brain stimulation. A. A 9-cm coil is placed on the scalp. A strong current in the coil creates a magnetic field which induces small currents in conductors in the cortex. B. The strength of the magnetic field decreases with distance from the coil. C. The time courses of the magnetic field and the induced currents. The time course of the induced current is the derivative of the magnetic field (Hess et al., 1987).

over the lateral frontal cortex (Maccabbee et al., 1988). The speech inhibition is best when the coil is tilted at an angle of 45 degrees away from the skull.

These localization and orientation effects of magnetic stimulation have not been explained neurally.

Stimulation and recording of pyramidal cells in motor cortex

To explain these transcranial stimulation results, the excitation of cortical cells must be reviewed. The large pyramidal cells (primarily in layer five) provide the descending outputs of the cerebral cortex. These cells can be activated directly by microstimulation of the axon hillock or by high-current anodal stimulation of the surface of the cortex (Phillips & Porter, 1977; Jankowska et al., 1975). These cells can also be activated indirectly by high-current stimulation of the cortex surface, presumably by stimulating interneurons in the cortex (Patton & Amassian, 1954; Phillips & Porter, 1977). The indirect activation is much more sensitive to asphyxia, cortical damage, or barbiturate anesthesia, as would be expected for synaptic transmission through the cortex.

Stimulation from the surface with a single 0.2-msec anodal pulse can evoke

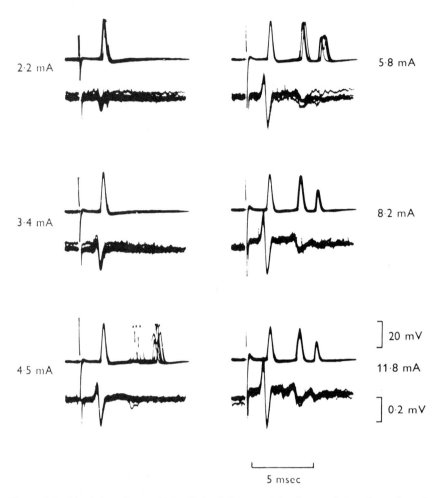

Figure 8-3. Stimulation of pyramidal cells by 0.2-ms anodal pulses applied to the surface of baboon motor cortex. The applied current is shown in the margins. Two recordings were made from the cervical spinal cord at each current: the upper records show the activity of a single corticospinal axon observed with a microelectrode and the lower records show the simultaneous activity recorded with a nearby large electrode from the cord surface. Each record shows about 10 superimposed tests. The first peak in each record shows the direct excitation of pyramidal cells, and the later peaks show the indirect excitation of pyramidal cells (Kernell & Wu, 1967).

several indirect action potentials. For example, as anodal currents increased from 3 to 12 mA, 1–4 indirect action potentials were added, each at a particular current (Figure 8-3) (Kernell & Wu, 1967). These action potentials were recorded in the cervical spinal cord. The indirect action potentials occurred very reliably, and each at a characteristic latency once the current threshold was exceeded.

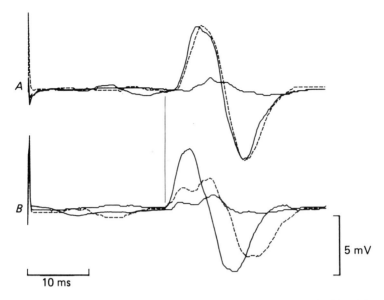

Figure 8-4. EMG response in a small muscle (abductor digiti minimi) of the right hand to magnetic (A) and electrical (B) stimulation at an intensity of 20 percent above threshold. The smallest responses are to stimulation while the muscle was relaxed, the dashed lines show the response while the muscle was contracted voluntarily at 10 percent of maximum, and the fastest responses are to stimulation while the muscle was contracted voluntarily at 25 percent of maximum. The latencies were shorter with electrical stimulation, but the amplitudes were greater with magnetic stimulation (Hess et al., 1987).

Mechanisms of magnetic and electrical transcranial stimulation

The short latencies of the responses (about 19–24 ms for hand muscles) to anodal electrical stimulation of the scalp are consistent with the direct activation of the fast corticospinal axons which synapse monosynaptically onto motoneurons in the primate spinal cord (Day et al., 1986; Hess et al., 1986). Most of this latency (about 13 msec) is due to the time from motor neuron activation to muscle response (Mills & Murray, 1986). The response to magnetic stimulation, however, has a 2-ms longer latency (Hess et al., 1987) (Figure 8-4). Therefore, magnetic stimulation is believed to be due to the activation of cortical interneurons, while anodal electrical stimulation is believed to be due primarily to the direct activation of pyramidal cell axons.

Two other properties of magnetic stimulation are accounted for by this hypothesis. First, weak electrical stimulation often produces a two-hump EMG response (Figure 8-4, dashed line). The 2-ms difference in latency between the two humps suggests that the first hump is due to direct pyramidal cell activation and the second hump is due to indirect activation. Second, the response to magnetic stimulation is facilitated by voluntary contraction of the hand muscles

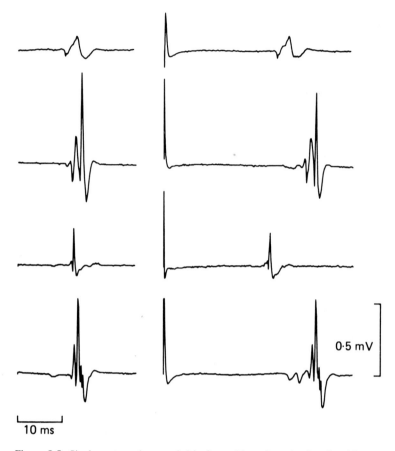

Figure 8-5. Single motor units recorded in four subjects from the first dorsal interosseous muscle of humans. The left figures show the units are active during minimal voluntary contraction of the muscle; the right figures show the activation of these same units by threshold magnetic stimulation of the cortex (Hess et al., 1987).

at much lower intensities than the response to electrical stimulation. This suggests that integration at the level of the cortex occurs as well as integration at the level of the spinal cord (Hess et al., 1987). Both electrical and magnetic stimulation are facilitated at the level of the spinal cord by a variety of reflex mechanisms.

Single motor units can be observed by recording with needle electrodes in the muscle (Figure 8-5). These units can be activated by weak voluntary contractions or by magnetic or electrical stimulation of the cortex. Often the unit that is most easily activated by a reflex or a voluntary contraction is the same unit that is most easily activated by cortical stimulation. These are not the fastest units, since the slower motor units have the lowest thresholds to synaptic activation, according to Henneman's size principle. Electrical stimulation of the motor nerves, however, activates the fastest motor units first, due to the low electrical thresholds of large fibers.

In conclusion, transcranial stimulation is a new, relatively safe tool to study the human brain. The differences between electrical and magnetic stimulation may prove to be useful in assessing cortical synaptic function. The mechanisms of action of induced currents in the cortex, however, are still poorly understood.

TRANSYNAPTIC COLLISION

In Chapters 4 through 7, double-pulse effects have been related to the refractory periods and conduction times of axons in a single bundle. In this section, asymmetric collision results that do not fit the axonal collision model are evaluated. A model of transynaptic collision is discussed where one electrode is presynaptic and the other is postsynaptic.

Model of transynaptic collision

Synaptic transmission is unlike axonal conduction. For example, synaptic transmission is probablistic and shows temporal and spatial summation (Sherrington, 1906). Also, transmission of excitation through the spinal cord occurs from dorsal roots to ventral roots, but not from ventral roots to dorsal roots; that is, synaptic transmission is one-way, not two-way. Therefore, symmetric collision cannot occur when stimulating across synapses.

Transynaptic collision is easily observed in monosynaptic stretch reflexes. Each strong presynaptic stimulus can evoke a large EPSP and at least one postsynaptic action potential. The first postsynaptic action potential can be blocked by stimulating the motor nerve at the appropriate time and evoking an antidromic action potential which then collides with the postsynaptic action potential. The conduction times of each of these action potentials and the synaptic transmission times are easily measured, and so the collision is easily arranged (Eccles, 1964).

A two-neuron model of transynaptic collision is shown in Figure 8-6. Assume that presynaptic action potentials evoked by C pulses at electrode A result in postsynaptic action potentials with some probability, p. A T pulse presented at electrode B evokes an antidromic action potential that can collide with one of those orthodromic action potentials on the postsynaptic axon between electrode B and the axon hillock (H). Collision cannot occur in presynaptic axons due to one-way synaptic transmission. (Interactions between potentials in the cell body and dendritic tree can occur, but these are beyond the scope of this model.)

For collision to occur, the C pulses must be presented early enough so that a presynaptic action potential can conduct the length of the presynaptic axon, transmit across the synapse, and initiate an action potential at H before the

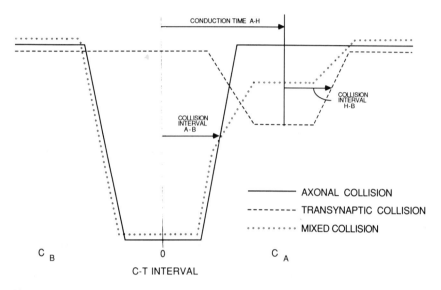

Figure 8-6. Model of transynaptic collision. Above: axonal collision can occur anywhere along the axon between the two stimulating electrodes. When stimulating across a synapse, however, collision can only occur on the postsynaptic axon between the spike initiating zone (H) and the postsynaptic electrode. Below: axonal collision (solid line) is symmetric around the C-T interval of 0. Transynaptic collision (dashed line) is symmetric around a positive C-T interval determined by the time to initiate an action potential at H. When both axonal and transynaptic collision occur (dotted line—mixed), both symmetric and asymmetric results are seen.

antidromic action potential has disappeared. The first C-T interval where collision occurs is the sum of the presynaptic conduction time and the synaptic delay, minus the postsynaptic collision interval. (This assumes that the time to initiate an action potential is the same for both neurons.) The postsynaptic collision interval is identical to the collision interval measured with electrodes at H and B. Collision will last until the postsynaptic action potential has conducted past B before the antidromic action potential is initiated. The last C-T interval where collision is observed is equal to the presynaptic conduction time plus the synaptic delay *plus* the postsynaptic collision interval. Therefore, transynaptic collision is symmetric around a positive C-T interval equal to the presynaptic conduction time plus the synaptic delay. The synaptic delay can be more variable than conduction times or collision intervals. The maximum percent collision will equal p.

In brain stimulation, pure transynaptic collision has never been reported. It is harder to match axons transynaptically, so that each presynaptic action potential results in a single transynaptic collision. Nonetheless, if a proportion of presynaptic action potentials are transmitted, then some transynaptic collision should occur. Also, the timing of transynaptic action potentials is harder to predict in the brain. If many axons and/or many synapses are involved, the results will become more variable due to the various refractory periods, conduction times, and synaptic delays involved, and the lower probabilities of transmission through more than one synapse.

Mixed axonal and transynaptic collision

Figure 8-7 shows the first examples of asymmetric collision. The two electrodes were in the anteromedial cortex and striatum. The response observed was the frequency threshold for contraversive circling in rats. Symmetric collision was seen for some electrode pairs (Panel C) at C-T intervals of 0.6 to 1.0 msec, with a slight rise at intervals from 1.0 to 10 msec. This suggests that mainly fast axons between the cortex and striatum mediate contraversive circling.

Asymmetric collision is seen in Panels A and B for two other electrode pairs. At C-T intervals from 1.0 to 4.0 msec, the two curves clearly diverge. That is, recovery was abrupt between 1.0 and 2.0 msec when the C pulses were presented via the striatal electrode, but recovery occurred much later (between 2.0 and 6.0 msec) when C pulses were presented via the cortical electrode.

Our interpretation of these results is that both axonal and transynaptic collision occurred. If both axonal and transynaptic collision occur, then a sharp symmetric rise should be seen as some C-T intervals and a slower asymmetric rise should be seen at other C-T intervals (Figure 8-6). According to this interpretation, symmetric collision of about 20 percent was seen at C-T intervals of 0.6 to 1.0 msec, at both low and high currents. This symmetric collision is attributable to direct activation of the fast axons between the cortex and striatum seen in Panel A.

The asymmetry observed at C-T intervals from 1.0 to 4.0 msec suggests that transynaptic circuits must be stimulated between the cortex and striatum as well as axonal circuits. The one-way conduction across the synapses must be from anterior to posterior, since the curve rose slower when the C pulses were delivered to the anterior electrode. The probability of transynaptic firing (p) must be high, since the 25 percent asymmetry observed at 2.0 msec was greater than the axonal collision. The conduction time plus synaptic delay on the presynaptic neurons must be near 2 msec on the average. The collision interval on the postsynaptic axons must be short (roughly 1 msec), since the asymmetry was clearly observed only at C-T intervals of 2.0 and 3.0 msec. The postsynaptic axons in this circuit must also be fast.

This interpretation of the cortex-striatum collision experiment is consistent with the studies of pyramidal cells discussed above. The symmetric collision is attributed to direct stimulation of the fast axons of pyramidal cells. The asymmetric collision is attributed to indirect stimulation of these same pyramidal cells 1 to 3 msec later than the direct stimulation. The indirect activation of

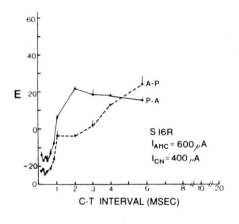

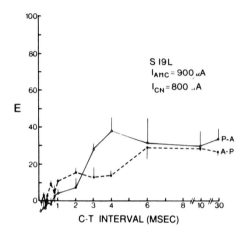

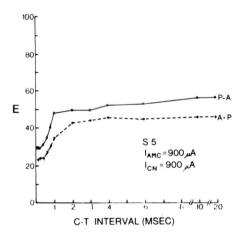

Figure 8-7. Collision tests between the anteromedial cortex and rostral striatum electrode sites where circling is evoked in rats. E is the same as in Chapter 7. Lower panel: symmetric collision suggests that fast axons between the cortex and striatum mediate circling. Upper panels: asymmetric collision in some sites suggest that transynaptic circuits from the cortex to rostral striatum also can produce circling (Yeomans & Buckenham, 1988).

pyramidal cells is reliable enough and at the right latencies to account for the asymmetric collision.

Refractory periods in the cortex

If each C pulse in cortex is stimulating both direct and indirect action potentials, then these pyramidal cells will be refractory to stimulation twice. They will be refractory during the direct firing (in the first millisecond) and again during all indirect firings (1–4 msec later). The refractory period curve will reflect these recovery times: (1) the refractory periods of the pyramidal cells, (2) the refractory periods of the interneurons responsible for the indirect activation of pyramidal cells, and (3) the recovery from collision between indirect and direct action potentials at C-T intervals 1–4 msec after the refractory period. Transynaptic collisions can block only one of the indirect action potentials, and so E should be reduced by no more than 50 percent due to transynaptic collisions.

Indeed, refractory period curves for circling in the anteromedial cortex often rise at very long C-T intervals. The first rise is in the 0.4 to 1.5 msec range, due to the refractory periods of pyramidal cells and perhaps interneurons. The second rise, which varies in size from 0 to 70 percent in different animals, is in the 2–4 msec range (Figure 8-8). This second rise, then, could be due to transynaptic collision, although the contribution of very long refractory period interneurons cannot be excluded. Similar rises at long C-T intervals have been observed in the medial prefrontal cortex for self-stimulation (Schenk & Shizgal, 1982), and in the striatum or superior colliculus for circling (Buckenham & Yeomans, 1988).

In conclusion, refractory period tests can be contaminated by transynaptic collision at long C-T intervals when both presynaptic and postsynaptic elements are stimulated by the electrode. Transynaptic collision can account for a shift in E of up to 50 percent, although much lower values would be expected in most cases.

Transynaptic summation

Another more speculative scenario is the *soma hypothesis* (Szabo, 1973). Stimulation near cell bodies could depolarize the soma, and this depolarization could sum with postsynaptic potentials. In this case, E values in the refractory period experiment would be higher at C-T intervals near the point of maximum asymmetry in the collision experiment. If the PSPs declined gradually over several milliseconds, however, this effect would simply counteract the transynaptic collision effect, and so would be hard to observe. I have not yet seen any good data for transynaptic summation.

CONCLUSIONS

Although double-pulse experiments on brain stem stimulation have fit the axonal model of refractory periods and collision, cortical stimulation experiments

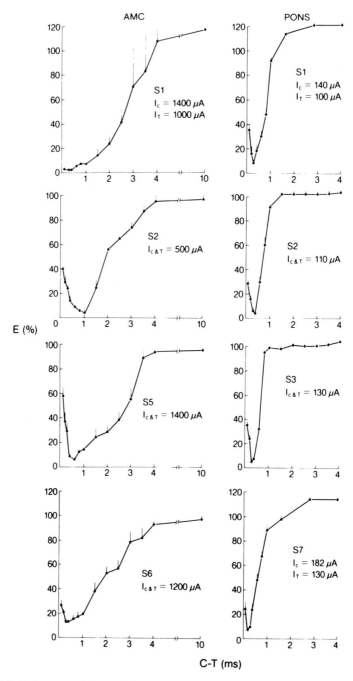

Figure 8-8. Refractory period tests in four anteromedial cortex sites where circling is evoked (left panels). The slow recovery at long C-T intervals may in part reflect transynaptic collision in the cortex rather than simple refractoriness (Tehovnik & Yeomans, 1987). Right panels show results from four pons sites in the same rats.

suggest that stimulation near high probability synapses can result in nonaxonal effects. Asymmetric collision between cortex and striatum seems to occur due to indirect activation of pyramidal cells. Recovery of refractory period curves at long C-T intervals could be due also, in part, to transynaptic collisions. These phenomena can be tested with the collision method, and so may open a new chapter in the study of synapses with double-pulse brain stimulation.

FURTHER READINGS

Dobelle, W.H., Mladejovsky, M.G., & Evans, J.R. "Braille" reading by a blind volunteer by visual cortex stimulation. *Nature,* 1976, *259,* 111–112.

Hess, C.W., Mills, K.R., & Murray, N.M.F. Responses in small hand muscles from magnetic stimulation of the human brain. *Journal of Physiology,* 1987, *388,* 397–419.

APPENDIX I

Paired-pulse Stimulation of Axon Bundles: Fields of Excitation

JOHN S. YEOMANS AND PATRICK GOEBEL

FIELDS OF EXCITATION FOR CATHODAL C AND T PULSES

The assumptions of the homogeneous bundle model of Chapter 3 are applied here. As discussed in Chapter 3 (Figure 3-6), the field of excitation for a single pulse is a circle in the cross section of the bundle at the electrode.

The excitation added by a T pulse is shown in Figure 6-5, as discussed in Chapter 6. On the left, the effects of delivering weaker T pulses is shown. Axons nearest the electrode fire twice at all C-T intervals longer than their ARPs. Farther from the electrode, recovery occurs later in the RRP. In their SNPs, these same axons can miss their second firing. Farther still from the electrode, recovery occurs in the SubNP. Therefore, when the C pulse is higher in current than the T pulse, the entire poststimulation excitability cycle is observable. In some more-distant axons, only C pulses produce excitation at all C-T intervals. Finally, axons which were not quite excited by the C pulses may produce local potentials that sum with T pulse excitation at very short C-T intervals.

The effects of stimulating with equal-current C and T pulses are shown in Figure 6-5, middle panel. The regions of recovery at the ARP and RRP or SubNP are the same as above. No recovery occurs during the SNP, however, since all axons excited by the C pulse are excited during their RRPs or ARPs by the equal-current T pulse. Axons not quite excited by the C pulse show local potential summation (LPS) at very short C-T intervals. The region of LPS is closer to the electrode than in the left panel, since the C pulse excites a smaller region on its own.

The effects of stimulating with higher-current T pulses is shown on the right. All axons excited by the C pulse recover at their ARPs. Outside of this region, the T pulse excites axons not quite excited by the C pulse at all C-T intervals. Farther from the electrode, LPS occurs at short C-T intervals. Therefore, after LPS subsides, all changes in excitation are due to recovery from the ARP.

EXCITATION OF SINGLE AXONS

The effects of stimulating a single axon with cathodal C and T pulses are shown quantitatively in Figure 6-5 and 6-6. The higher-current pulses are 1.5 times the lower- and equal-current pulses in these graphs. Although the ratio 1.5 is shown here, calculation of these graphs for any ratio, X, can be made by substituting X wherever 1.5 is shown. These are plotted in the excitability form with I_o/I on the vertical axis and C-T interval on the horizontal axis as in Figure 6-1. Similar curves plotted as I/I_o are found in Yeomans (1979).

The number of action potentials at each C-T interval is shown in Figure 6-6. Since I is proportional to the number of axons recruited (Chapter 3), the relative number of axons recruited is calculated at each C-T interval by the height of each region times the number of C's and T's in the region. Since more current is delivered in the unequal-current-pulses conditions, the total number of action potentials is greater in those conditions. The LPS curve falls faster using higher current C pulses. The absolute fall during LPS and the absolute rise during the poststimulation excitability cycle (PSEC) is essentially the same in all curves, however.

FIELDS OF EXCITATION FOR ANODAL C OR T PULSES

The effects of two anodal pulses are the same as two cathodal pulses, except that more current in required to produce comparable excitation in the anodal case. A single anodal pulse is useful, however, because it reverses LPS, thereby allowing complete separation of refractory period and LPS effects (Chapters 5 and 6; Yeomans et al., 1979). Strong anodal pulses, however, can produce depolarizations to threshold at more distant sites, and hence refractory period effects. Figure A-1 (upper panel) shows the regions of excitation for an anodal C and a cathodal T pulse, and a cathodal C pulse followed by an anodal T pulse. The pulses are of equal current, and it is assumed that the anodal pulse requires 2 times as much current as the cathodal pulse to produce excitation. The effects on a single axon are shown below.

Using one anodal pulse, the number of action potentials increases at C-T intervals in the LPS range (Figure A-2). At C-T intervals in the refractory period range, the number of action potentials also increases. The anodal pulses act like weaker cathodal pulses, and therefore the fields and number of action potentials are comparable to the unequal-current cathodal conditions.

The dotted line shows the results when a cathodal C pulse is followed by an anodal T pulse. In this case, LPS is reduced at the shortest C-T intervals. Only equal-current pulses are shown here, but the effects of unequal-current, anodal-cathodal combinations are easily calculated.

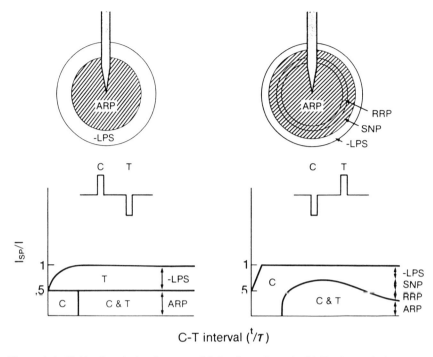

Figure A-1. Fields of excitation for an anodal C pulse and a cathodal T pulse, and vice versa. Above, the fields of excitation in a cross section of the bundle of axons at the electrode; below, excitability of a single axon at different C-T intervals.

FIELDS OF EXCITATION WHEN C AND T PULSES ARE DELIVERED VIA SEPARATE ELECTRODES

Stimulation through two electrodes is useful for defining the size of the field of excitation, the so-called current–distance relationship, or for tracing the trajectory of axons and determining their conduction velocities (Chapter 7).

When two electrodes are placed in a bundle in the same transverse plane, the fields of excitation change as a function of interelectrode distance $(2d)$. Five different distances are shown for equal current C and T pulses in Figure A-3. The effects of current are not considered separately here, because the same fields result when I/d^2 is held constant.

When $d=$ infinity, two separate circles of excitation occur. As the electrodes approach one another, LPS is added in ovals slightly larger than the circles, elongated toward the other electrode (Figure A-3A). These two fields of LPS just touch when $d=2^{1/2}r$, at a C-T interval of 0 (Figure A-3B). When $d=r$, a second firing occurs during the SNP for axons near the edge of the region of C pulse firings (Figure A-3C). When $d=.9r$, RRP and SubNP regions are added (Figure A-3D). When $d=.5r$, an ARP region is added (Figure A-3E). The

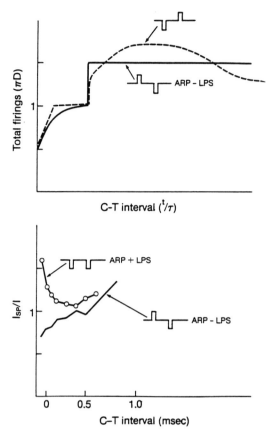

Figure A-2. Effects of anodal C pulses on behavior. Above, predicted total number of firings from Figure A-1. Below, results of a behavioral experiment (MFB self-stimualtion) comparing cathodal pulse pairs to pairs with an anodal C pulse followed by a cathodal T pulse (Yeomans et al., 1979).

condition $d=0$ (Figure A-3G) is the equal-current, one-electrode condition described in Figures 6-5 and 6-6 above, and so the SNP region disappears. The regions of the PSEC are determined by the radial distance from the T electrode, as it intersects with the circle around the C electrode.

EQUATIONS FOR PSEC FIELDS

The fields of excitation for the PSEC are easily described mathematically, since the PSEC is independent of the intensity of the above-threshold C pulse. Therefore, the fields are determined by the intersection of two circles: one defined by the radial distance from the electrode delivering the C pulse *(r)*, and the second defined by the radial distance from the electrode delivering the T pulse *(r2)*. The general equation for two intersecting circles is:

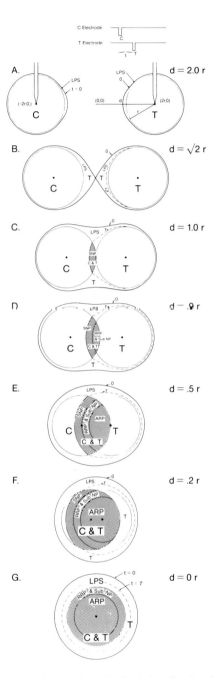

Figure A-3. Fields of excitation for two-electrode stimulation, C pulses through the left electrode and T pulses through the right electrode. Going from top to bottom, as the electrodes move together (or current increases), first LPS, then SNP, then RRP and SubNP, then ARP effects occur. The ovals marked 0 show the fields of LPS at a C-T interval of 0; the dashed curves marked τ show the fields of LPS at a C-T interval equal to the time constant of the axons. The variable d is half the interelectrode distance. The variable r is the radius of the single-pulse fields in panel A.

$$A = [r2^2 \cos^{-1}(y/r2) + r^2 \cos^{-1}((d-y)/r)] - d(r2^2 - y^2)^{1/2}$$

where

$$y = (d^2 + r2^2 - r^2)/2d$$

A is the area of intersection of the two circles (Yeomans et al., 1984).

When equal-current C and T pulses are presented, the number of action potentials depends on C-T interval and interelectrode distance (Figure A-4). If the interelectrode distance is infinite, the number of excitations per pair at all C-T intervals is equal to the area of the two circles times the density of axons, or:

$$N \text{ firings/pair} = 2\pi r^2 D$$

When the interelectrode distance is 0, the number of firings/pair is $\pi r^2 D$ inside the ARP and $2\pi r^2 D$ outside the RRP. If r is set equal to 1, the equation for the total number of firings/pair is:

$$N \text{ firings/pair} = D\ (2\pi - A_{r2=1} + A_{r2})$$

where $A_{r2=1}$ is the area of intersection when the radius of the T pulse excitation is the same as the C pulse excitation, and A_{r2} is the area of intersection when T pulse excitation can vary due to the C-T interval and PSEC (ARP, RRP, SNP or SubNP). This is plotted as a function of d/r in Figure A-4. This variable measures the interelectrode distance in units of the circle radius. The effect of changing the current, or the threshold of the axons, is to alter r. Values for unequal currents can be calculated from equations 1 and 2.

$r2$ is chosen to be equal to 0.8 at the beginning of the RRP and peak of the SubNP, and 1.2 at the peak of the SNP. The family of curves is shown, however, so that other values can be calculated for any point on the PSEC by $I = Kr^2$. These results are plotted as a function of C-T interval in Figure A-5.

EQUATIONS FOR LOCAL POTENTIAL SUMMATION FIELDS

The fields of excitation for LPS are more complicated, however, since they depend on the distances from both electrodes jointly. The local potential is proportional to the current density, and current density falls off as the inverse square. Therefore, when the two pulses are delivered simultaneously, the LPS curve is the locus of points for which

$$(r/r1)^2 + (r/r2)^2 = 1,$$

where r is the radius of excitation for a C pulse, $r1$ is the distance from the electrode delivering the C pulse to the axon, and $r2$ is the distance from the T

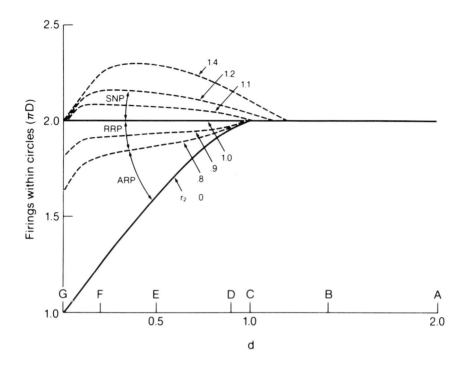

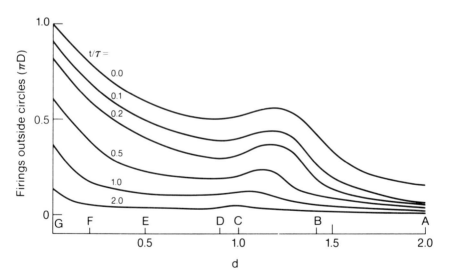

Figure A-4. Total firings for two-electrode stimulation, shown as a function of interelectrode distance. A. Total firings within the single-pulse circles of Figure A-3. The dashed lines show the added T pulse firings as the radius of the field increases from 0 to 1.4 radii away from the T electrode. B. Total firings outside the single-pulse circles, due to the added effects of LPS. As the C-T interval (measured in units of t/τ) increases, the added firings decrease.

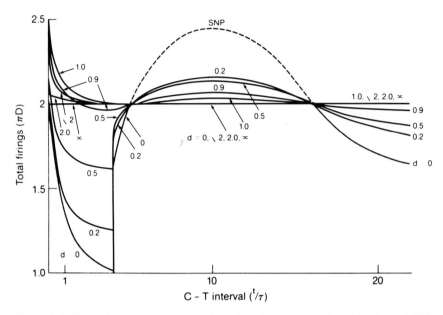

Figure A-5. Total firings for two-electrode stimulation, shown as a function of C-T interval. Values of d from 2 to 0 are shown. The percent refractoriness decreases as the interelectrode distance increases. The dashed line labeled SNP shows that the SNP is cut off when $d=0$.

electrode to the axon. The field in which excitation occurs at a C-T interval of 0 is described by the equation:

$$[(x^2+y^2)-(r^2-(d/2)^2)]^2=r^4+x^2d^2$$

where the electrodes are located at $x=\pm d/2$. When d is large relative to r, this equation approaches two circles centered at the electrodes. When d is small relative to r, this equation approaches a circle with radius $2^{(1/2)}r$. This equation is a variation on the equation for the ovals of Cassini (Beyer, 1981). When $d=2^{(3/2)}r$, this equation reduces to:

$$(x^2+y^2)^2=r^4\,(3x^2-y^2)$$

This curve is a *two-leaved rose* (Figure A-3A) related to the lemniscate of Bernoulli intersecting the origin at 60°.

When the C pulse is delivered before the T pulse, the local potential due to the C pulse declines exponentially. Therefore, at threshold, the locus of points becomes:

$$e^{(-t/\tau)}\,(r/r1)^2+(r/r2)^2=1$$

where t is the C-T interval, and τ is the time constant of LPS decay. The general description of the field excitation for LPS, then, is

$$e^{-t/\tau}[x^2 + y^2 + (d/2)^2]^2 - r^2(e^{-t/\tau} + 1)[x^2 + y^2 + (d/2)^2] = dr^2x(e^{-t/\tau} - 1)$$

This field is not symmetrical at ($0 > t <$ infinity) because more decay occurs for local potentials near the C electrode than near the T electrode. In Figure A-3, the spatial fields of excitation for LPS are shown for two cases, $t = 0$ and $t = \tau$.

This sequence of effects cannot be graphed spatially and temporally in two dimensions (as in Figure 6-6 for one electrode), since the spatial dimension is not radially symmetrical and therefore requires two dimensions alone. The total number of action potentials can be calculated from the equations above, however, as a function of C-T interval and interelectrode distance. The seven inter-electrode distances ($d = 0$, $.2r$, $.5r$, $.9r$, r, $2^{(1/2)}$ r, and $2r$) of Figure A-3 are shown in Figure A-5.

These equations were integrated numerically. In general, the duration and amount of LPS decreases as d increases. The relationship is not monotonic, however, since LPS is slightly better at $d = r$ (when the fields just touch) than at $d = .9r$, or $1.5r$ (Figure A-4).

CONCLUSIONS

The effects of stimulation with two electrodes are much more complicated than described previously (Fouriezos & Wise, 1984; Yeomans et al., 1986). LPS can be appreciable when pulses are presented simultaneously, but is much smaller at time τ. As interelectrode distance decreases, SNP effects are observed first, followed by RRP and ARP effects. ARP effects contribute last, and more slowly than SNP and RRP effects. The ratio d/r must be less than 0.5 before ARP effects are larger than SNP and RRP effects together for the PSEC curve shown. SNP effects are likely to make a large contribution at 5.0 msec when overlap in fields is partial.

These results are applicable to collision experiments if the axons are assumed to be continuous and parallel between the two electrodes (see Figure 7-10). The misalignment of the two electrodes in the bundle is simply the interelec-trode distance $(2d)$ calculated from Figure A-5. The conduction time between electrodes must be added to all times. Also, no LPS fields occur in collision experiments when the electrodes are far apart.

LPS can occur in the collision experiment if the electrodes are close together or the currents are high. LPS depends not on the distance between electrodes in the plane transverse to the bundle, but on the actual distance between elec-trodes (including the distance in the direction longitudinal to the bundle). We have not attempted to model this, however, since the mathematics is difficult and the difference between longitudinal and transverse impedance in a bundle becomes critical in the calculation.

APPENDIX II

Practical Notes for Brain Stimulators

In this appendix, some practical problems for electrical brain stimulation are discussed, including stimulators, electrodes, surgery, and histology. In many cases, the specific gadgets or practices preferred here will become dated as new equipment or tricks of the trade become available. Although this chapter is therefore the most expendable, it may serve as a guide to check or improve on techniques. My own experience is limited to stimulating rats using electrodes of 10 to 400 μm diameter.

STIMULATORS

Most stimulators deliver constant-current pulses, or have an attachment for delivering constant-current pulses. Unfortunately, only one of the commercially available stimulators (made by Stimtek, Arlington, MA) shunts the electrodes to ground between pulses, to the best of my knowledge. For other commercial stimulators, pulses should be delivered in a biphasic or capacitance-coupled waveform to prevent polarization of the electrodes. If you prefer, good stimulators can easily be built from integrated circuits (Mundl, 1980; Doty & Bartlett, 1981; Gallistel, 1981). These devices can be interfaced to microcomputers so that programs can be written to automatically determine stimuli. One stimulator allows automatic control of four independent outputs from a single Apple 2E computer (Campbell et al., 1985). The computer program was designed for testing self-stimulating animals, and for determining required frequency repeatedly—for example, to test the effects of drugs on self-stimulation.

ELECTRODES AND LESIONS

The ideal material for electrodes is stable chemically when current is passed, and produces minimal damage to brain tissue. Platinum wire is the most stable chemically and produces minimal damage, and is therefore relatively safe for long-term studies (Doty & Bartlett, 1981). Platinum is soft, however, and so must be hardened with 10–20 percent iridium to allow accurate placement of depth electrodes. Platinum is the material of choice for studies in which safety is more important than cost, as in permanent human implants (Pudenz et al.,

1975), or in studies which use long duration or anodal waveforms (e.g., Matthews, 1977).

Stainless steel is still the most often-used and readily available material. It is hard and durable. Investigators using anodal stimulation should not use stainless steel, since iron is deposited from the anode.

In general, lesions depend on the total charge independent of pulse duration. For example, lesions produced by platinum electrodes are determined by the total charge in each waveform (Pudenz et al., 1977), possibly because the total charge determines the volume of hydrogen gas production, according to Faraday's First Law of Electrochemistry. Hydrogen bubble formation begins at 1.7 V (Glasstone, 1946) in saline using platinum electrodes and at slightly higher voltages using stainless steel electrodes. The quantity of iron deposition with stainless steel is also related to the total charge emitted from the anodal electrode.

Excitation, however, depends on the distribution of charge over time. The charge required for excitation increases as the pulse duration increases due to the strength-duration relationship. Therefore, the excitation/lesion ratio is greatest for short-duration pulses.

The critical test for functional damage due to brain stimulation is not bubble production, iron deposition, or even tissue damage, but whether function is altered by the electrodes over time. The best evidence for proper stimulation methods is the stability of thresholds over time (e.g., Swadlow, 1982).

When 60 Hz sine-waves are used, progressive damage with stainless steel electrodes is common. Each cycle delivers 8.3 msec anodal pulses. Anodal pulses of 5 msec or greater can severely increase thresholds and damage tissue, even at currents below 100 μA, in my experience.

Chronic electrodes can be purchased in platinum or stainless steel for monopolar or bipolar stimulation, already insulated and with convenient connectors. I prefer stainless steel insect pins (size 00 or 0) which have strong shafts (254-μm or 350-μm diameter) and a smoothly tapered tip that passes easily through rat dura or other hard tissue without bending. The tip is tapered over the last 2-mm of length to a tip smaller than 10 μm in diameter. The tip is easy to shape by rubbing on fine sandpaper. The diameter of the tip is easily controlled by the duration and intensity of the abrasion. Insect pins, however, must be soldered to a connector and insulated.

The population of stimulated neurons depends on the tip surface area. In general, to stimulate very few neurons using currents of 0.1 to 10 μA, microelectrodes with tip diameters of 2 to 20 μm must be used. To stimulate large numbers of axons using currents of 100–1,000 μA, macroelectrodes with tip diameters of 100–300 μm should be used. Mainly low threshold elements (large myelinated fibers and initial segments) are likely to be excited in either case. To stimulate more unmyelinated fibers, smaller tips or higher currents must be used. As a rule of thumb, the diameter of the hemispherical electrode tip should be at least one-fifth the maximum diameter of the field to be stimulated. In this case, the current density at the tip is roughly 50 times the current density at the edge of the field, so this should not be exceeded.

The tip exposure is made by scraping insulation off the tip. We use hemispherically shaped tips to eliminate jagged edges or points that might alter current density. Although the theoretical surface area of a hemisphere is $2\pi r^2$, the effective surface area for the neurons is larger, due to the added distance for the glial cells surrounding the tip. The glial sheath is thickest from a few days to a few weeks after surgery, then shrinks substantially.

The electrical surface area, which is much larger than the area of exposure to the axons, is determined by the roughness of the metal surface and is measured by the impedance in saline. Impedance should vary from 1 KOhm (large tip) to 500 KOhms (small tip). Microelectrodes are usually in the low MOhm range.

Movable electrodes can be made from small screw devices designed to fit on the head of moving animals. The best of these for rats are precisely machined and designed, and weigh as little as 0.26 g (Miliaressis & Gratton, 1981; Kinetrode, Ottawa, Ontario). Each 360 degree turn results in a 320 μm lowering of the electrode, but smaller steps can be made by smaller turns.

If many electrodes must be lowered, it is often easier to fix the electrodes together beforehand. Gallistel (1981) suggests drilling holes stereotaxically in a wood or plastic block placed in the stereotaxic instrument. The electrodes can then be fixed in place with dental cement and removed from the block for surgery.

Small receivers are now available for delivering stimulation by radio signals rather than wires to monkeys and humans, or even some small animals (Delgado, 1981). This eliminates the problems of wires between stimulator and animal, but requires batteries.

DURABLE IMPLANTS

Implants can come loose in long-term experiments where animals can scratch at, pull, or damage the implants. The loss of a subject that has been studied for weeks or months can be disastrous to an experiment.

First, it is essential that sterile surgical procedures be used. The electrodes themselves can carry infections which cause abcesses near the electrode tips. The wound should be sutured closed, so that the head and electrode cap are not routes for infection. Infections can form under the cap and lift up the implant, or around the screws in the skull (especially if these are not sterilized). We routinely give penicillin and an analgesic after surgery.

Second, the security of the implant rests on the security of the skull screws, not on the contact of the cement with the skull. In fact, Richard Miselis of the University of Pennsylvania Veterinary School recommends that the periosteum, the membrane over the cranial surface, be left intact over as much of the cranium as possible with the cement above. This keeps the bone healthy and resists growth or infection in the damaged and exposed skull. The small islands of exposed bone where the screws are to be lowered must be dried thoroughly (for example, by placing a drop of epinephrine to reduce blood flow) to a white color before drilling holes. The drill holes should be angled inward about 20 degrees from vertical. Each screw, then, will enter at a different angle, so that even if the screws are loose the implant cannot be raised out in any one direction. The screws should be lowered in at exactly the same angle as the holes so that the holes are not enlarged.

The implant should fit close to the skull. If the electrodes stick out, the animal will grab and pull at them. Also, if the dental cement is not formed smoothly on the skull, the animal can grab underneath this or at one of the protrusions. Most animals accept a smooth, flat implant in a short time, however. Fresh blood around the implant implies a loose implant or an open wound. The wound should be treated with antiseptic and allowed to heal.

HISTOLOGY

The depth of the stimulation site is hard to determine, since the tip can damage or tear the brain during removal. To keep from damaging the tip site, the electrodes should be raised through the same track that they were lowered. The stimulation site can be identified if a tiny lesion (anodal d.c. current of 0.2 mA for 10–30 seconds) is made near the tip at the time of sacrifice. If stainless steel electrodes are used, the iron deposits can be stained with a ferricyanide solution by soaking the brain overnight in a solution of 3 percent ferricyanide, 3 percent ferrocyanide, and 0.5 percent trichloroacetic acid.

After sectioning and mounting on slides, there are many choices of stains. Cell body stains, such as Thionin (bluish purple) or cresyl violet (Wolf, 1971), help locate the stimulation site due to glial cell growth around the tip. Since electrical stimulation works mainly on myelinated axons, some prefer to use a myelin stain, such as the Weil-Weigert method. The Klüver-Barrera method stains both axons and cells, so it is ideal if mastered.

If the cells of origin are known, the best axon stain is the PHA-L method of Gerfen and Sawchenko (1984). PHA-L is taken up by cells near the injection site and transported orthogradely in the axons. The axons can be traced easily for many millimeters. This method allows one to estimate the diameter of large axons passing by an electrode from a particular site, and also to differentiate axon terminals from axons of passage. It is difficult, however, to get good results reliably with this technique.

Two methods for measuring neural activity anatomically are the ^{14}C-deoxy-glucose method of Sokoloff (Kennedy et al., 1975), and the cytochrome oxi-dase method of Wong-Riley (1979). The deoxyglucose method relies on the fact that active neurons take up more glucose than inactive neurons. Deoxyglu-cose is a glucose analog that cannot be metabolized and is therefore trapped. The uptake of deoxyglucose can be measured by injecting the animals with ^{14}C-deoxyglucose, waiting 30 minutes to an hour for the deoxyglucose to be taken up into brain cells, removing and sectioning the brain, and placing the

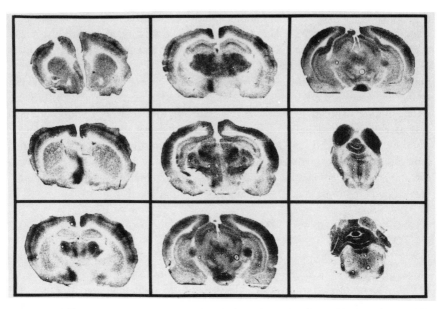

Figure A-6. ^{14}C-deoxyglucose radiograph of rat brain section, taken from self-stimulating rat with electrode in left preoptic area. Increased uptake is shown by increased darkness. Note the increased uptake of tracer for about 1 mm around the electrode. The rat bar pressed at a rate of 50 per second, for 500-msec trains of 500-μA stimulation, 100 Hz, 0.1-msec pulses, for 30 minutes following the injection.

dried brain slices against X-ray film for a week. The result is an autoradiograph which shows regional brain metabolic activity in the time period after the injection.

An autoradiograph taken from a rat which self-stimulated through an MFB electrode following the injection is shown in Figure A-6 (Yeomans et al., 1978). Darker areas represent more deoxyglucose, as shown by the radiographic standards on the right. In the left hypothalamus, where the stimulating electrode was placed, the region around the electrode and along the MFB is much darker than the opposite, unstimulated side of the brain. The lack of effect (or bilateral effects) in other structures is harder to interpret, however, since the sensitivity of the method varies from structure to structure (Gallistel, 1981).

The cytochrome oxidase method stains mitochondria, the energy-producing structures of cells: when more energy is used, more of the cytochromes are stained. The advantage of this technique over deoxyglucose is that the stain is attached to the structures, and so can be visualized to the limits of light microscopy in the tissue. The spatial resolution is therefore near 1 μm, whereas ^{14}C localization has a resolution nearer 50 μm, unless more advance procedures (thin sections, dipping in photographic emulsion, and fixing, or ^{3}H autoradiograph) are used. Cytochrome oxidase, however, may be less sensitive to brain activity changes than deoxyglucose.

References

Asanuma, H. Microstimulation technique. In *Electrical Stimulation Research Techniques*. M.M. Patterson and R.P. Kesner (Eds.). New York: Academic Press, 1981. pp. 61–70.

Asanuma, H., & Rosen, I. Topographical organization of cortical efferent zones projecting to distal forelimb muscles in the monkey. *Experimental Brain Research*, 1972, *14*, 243–256.

Asanuma, H., Arnold, A., & Zarzecki, P. Further study on the excitation of pyramidal tract cells by intracortical microstimulation. *Experimental Brain Research*, 1976, *26*, 443–461.

Barrett, E.F., & Barrett, J.N. Intracellular recording from vertebrate myelinated axons: Mechanism of the depolarizing afterpotential. *Journal of Physiology (London)*, 1982, *323*, 117–144.

Barry, F.E., Walter, M.S., & Gallistel, C.R. On the optimal pulse duration in electrical stimulation of the brain. *Physiology and Behavior*, 1974, *12*, 749–754.

Baylor, D.A., Matthews, G., & Yau, K.-W. Two components of electrical dark noise in toad retinal rod outer segments. *Journal of Physiology (London)*, 1980, *309*, 591–621.

Bean, C.P. A theory of microstimulation of myelinated fibers. Appendix to C. Abzug, M. Maeda, B.W. Peterson, & V.J. Wilson. Cervical branching of lumbar vestibulospinal axons. *Journal of Physiology (London)*, 1974, *243*, 499–522.

BeMent, S.L. Single myelinated peripheral nerve fibers—anatomic and electrophysiologic studies relevant to conduction velocity and fiber diameter histogram prediction from surface recorded potentials. In *Conduction Velocity Distributions: A Population Approach to Electrophysiology of Nerve*, L.J. Dorfman, K.L. Cummins, & L.L. Leifer (Eds.). New York: Alan R. Liss, 1981. pp. 33–55.

BeMent, S.L., & Ranck, J.B. Jr. A quantitative study of electrical stimulation of central myelinated fibers with monopolar electrodes. *Experimental Neurology*, 1969, *24*, 147–170. (a)

BeMent, S.L., & Ranck, J.B. Jr. A model for electrical stimulation of central myelinated fibers with monopolar electrodes. *Experimental Neurology*, 1969, *24*, 171–186. (b)

Bender, M.B. (ed). *The Oculomotor System*. New York: Harper & Row, 1964.

Beyer, W.H. *CRC Standard Mathematical Tables, 26th Edition*. Boca Raton: CRC Press, 1981. p. 271.

Bielajew, C., & Fouriezos, G. Post-stimulation excitability of mediodorsal thalamic self-stimulation. *Behavioural Brain Research*, 1985, *17*, 97–102.

Bielajew, C., Jordan, C., Ferme-Enright, J., & Shizgal, P. Refractory periods and anatomical linkage of the substrates for lateral hypothalamic and periaqueductal gray self-stimulation. *Physiology and Behavior*, 1981, *27*, 95–104.

Bielajew, C., Jurgens, S., & Fouriezos, G. The effect of pulse duration on refractory periods of neurons mediating brain-stimulation reward. *Behavioural Brain Research*, 1987 *24*, 233–241.

Bielajew, C., LaPointe, M., Kiss, I., & Shizgal, P. Absolute and relative refractory periods of the substrates for lateral hypothalamic and ventral midbrain self-stimulation. *Physiology and Behavior*, 1982, *28*, 125–132.

Bielajew, C., & Shizgal, P. Dissociation of the substrates for medial forebrain bundle self-stimulation and stimulation-escape using a two-electrode stimulation technique. *Physiology and Behavior*, 1980, *25*, 707–711.

Bielajew, C., & Shizgal, P. Behaviorally derived measures of conduction velocity in the substrate for rewarding medial forebrain bundle stimulation. *Brain Research*, 1982, *237*, 107–119.

Bielajew, C., & Shizgal, P. Evidence implicating descending fibers in self-stimulation of the medial forebrain bundle in rats. *Journal of Neuroscience*, 1986, *6*, 919–929.

Bowe, C.M., Kocsis, J.D., & Waxman, S.G. Association between the depolarizing afterpotential and the supernormal period in myelinated fibers. *Society for Neuroscience Abstracts*, 1985, *11*, 1184.

Boyd, I.A. The relation between conduction velocity and diameter for the three groups of efferent fibers in nerves to mammalian skeletal muscle. *Journal of Physiology (London)*, 1964, *175*, 33–35.

Boye, S., & Rompre, P.-P. Evidence for a direct link between reward-relevant neurons in the ventral tegmental area-posterior hypothalamus and the medial mesencephalon. *Society for Neuroscience Abstracts*, 1987, *13*, 1544.

Brindley, G.S. Electroejaculation: its technique, neurological implications and uses. *Journal of Neurology, Neurosurgery and Psychiatry*, 1981, *44*, 9–18.

Brindley, G.S. Effects of electrical stimulation of the visual cortex. *Human Neurobiology*, 1982, *1*, 281–283.

Brindley, G.S., & Craggs, M.D. A technique for anodally blocking large nerve fibres through chronically implanted electrodes. *Journal of Neurology, Neurosurgery and Psychiatry*, 1980, *43*, 1083–1090.

Brindley, G.S., & Lewin, W. The sensations produced by electrical stimulation of the visual cortex. *Journal of Physiology (London)*, 1968, *196*, 479–493.

Brindley, G.S., & Rushton, D.N. Implanted stimulators of the visual cortex as visual prosthetic devices. *Transactions of the American Academy of Ophthalmology and Otolaryngology*, 1974, *78*, OP741–745.

Bruce, C.J., Goldberg, M.E., Bushnell, M.C., & Stanton, G.B. Primate frontal eye fields II. Physiological and anatomical correlates of electrically evoked eye movements. *Journal of Neurophysiology*, 1985, *54*, 701–734.

Buckenham, K.E., & Yeomans, J.S. An uncrossed tectopontine pathway mediates ipsiversive turning. In preparation.

Bunney, B.S., Walters, J.R., Roth, R.H., & Aghajanian, G.K. Dopaminergic neurons: effects of antipsychotic drugs and amphetamine on single cell activity. *Journal of Pharmacology and Experimental Therapeutics*, 1973, *185*, 560–571.

Burne, R.A., Azizi, S.A., Mihailoff, G.A., & Woodward, D.J. The tectopontine projection in the rat with comments on visual pathways to the basilar pons. *Journal of Comparative Neurology*, 1981, *202*, 287–307.

Campbell, K.A., Evans, G., & Gallistel, C.R. A microcomputer-based method for physiologically interpretable measurement of the rewarding efficacy of brain stimulation. *Physiology and Behavior,* 1985, *35,* 395–403.

Cheney, P.D., & Fetz, E.E. Comparable patterns of muscle facilitation evoked by individual corticomotoneuronal (CM) cells and by single intracortical microstimuli in primates: evidence for functional groups of CM cells. *Journal of Neurophysiology,* 1985, *53,* 786–804.

Chu, N., & Bloom, F.E. Norepinephrine-containing neurons: changes in spontaneous discharge patterns during sleeping and waking. *Science,* 1973, *179,* 908.,

Corbett, D., LaFerriere, A., & Milner, P. Elimination of medial prefrontal cortex self-stimulation following transection of efferents to the sulcal cortex in the rat. *Physiology and Behavior,* 1982, *29,* 425–431.

Corbett, D., Stellar, J.R., Stinus, L., Kelley, A., & Fouriezos, G. Time course of alpha-flupenthixol explains "response artifacts" of neuroleptic action on brain reward. *Science,* 1982, *16,* 1251–1252.

Davis M. The mammalian startle response. In *Neural Mechanisms of Startle Behavior,* R.C. Eaton (ed). New York: Plenum Press, 1984, pp. 287–351.

Davis, M., Gendelman, D. S., Tischler, M.D., & Gendelman, P.M. A primary acoustic startle circuit: Lesion and stimulation studies. *Journal of Neuroscience,* 1982, *2* 791–805.

Day, B.L., Dick, J.P.R., Marsden, C.D., & Thompson, P.D. Differences between electrical and magnetic stimulation of the human brain. *Journal of Physiology* (London), 1986, *378,* 36P.

Dean, P., Redgrave, P., Sahibzada, N., & Tsuji, K. Head and body movements produced by electrical stimulation of superior colliculus in rats: Effects of interruption of crossed tectoreticulospinal pathway. *Neuroscience,* 1986, *19,* 367–380.

Delgado, J.M.R. Depth stimulation of the brain. In *Electrical Stimulation Research Methods,* M.M. Patterson and R.P. Kesner (Eds.). New York: Academic Press, 1981. pp. 105–140.

Dennis, S.G., Yeomans, J.S., & Deutsch, J.A. Adaptation of aversive brain stimulation. III. Excitability characteristics of behaviorally relevant substrates. *Behavioral Biology,* 1976, *18,* 531–544.

Deutsch, J.A. Behavioral measurement of the neural refractory period and its application to intracranial self-stimulation. *Journal of Comparative and Physiological Psychology,* 1964, *58,* 1–9.

Deutsch, J.A., & Collins, R. Facilitation as a function of temporal spacing in intracranial self-stimulation. *Nature,* 1965, *208,* 592–593.

Dobelle, W.H.., Mladejovsky, M.G., & Evans, J.R. "Braille" reading by a blind volunteer by visual cortex stimulation. *Nature,* 1976, *259,* 111–112.

Dorfman, L.J., Cummins, K.L. & Leifer, L.J. (Eds.) *Conduction Velocity Distributions: A Population Approach to Electrophysiology of Nerve.* New York: Liss, 1982.

Doty, R. W., & Bartlett, J.R. Stimulation of the brain via metallic electrodes. In *Electrical Stimulation Research Techniques,* M.M. Patterson and R.P. Kesner (Eds.). New York: Academic Press, 1981. pp. 71–103.

Durivage, A., & Miliaressis, E. Dissociation of MFB self-stimulation and exploration fibers using the collision technique. *Society for Neuroscience Abstracts,* 1983, *9,* 977.

Durivage, A., & Miliaressis, E. Anatomical dissociation of the substrates of medial forebrain bundle self-stimulation and exploration. *Behavioral Neuroscience,* 1987, *101,* 57–61.

Eccles, J.C. *The Physiology of Synapses*. New York: Academic Press, 1964.

Ellard, C.G., & Goodale, M.A. The role of the predorsal bundle in head and body movements elicited by electrical stimulation of the superior colliculus in the Mongolian gerbil. *Experimental Brain Research*, 1986, *64*, 421–433.

Eng, D.L., & Kocsis, J.D. Changes in membrane depolarization and extracellular potassium concentration during the supernormal period of turtle olfactory nerve. *Society for Neuroscience Abstracts*, 1985, *11*, 1185.

Erlanger, J., & Gasser, H.S. *Electrical Signs of Nervous Activity*. London: Oxford University Press, 1937.

Evans, J. R., Gordon, J., Abramov, I., Mladejovsky, M.G., & Dobelle, W.H. Brightness of phosphenes elicited by electrical stimulation of human visual cortex. *Sensory Processes*, 1979, *3*, 82–94.

Ferrier, D. *The Functions of the Brain*. London: Smith Edler, 1876 (1st ed.) 1886 (2nd ed.).

Foerster, A.P. Spontaneous regeneration of cut axons in adult rat brain. *Journal of Comparative Neurology*, 1982, *210*, 335–356.

Foerster, O. Zur operativen Behandlung der Epilepsie. *Deutsche Zeitschrift für Nervenheilkunde*, 1926, *89*, 137–147.

Fouriezos, G., & Wise, R.A. Current-distance relation for rewarding brain stimulation. *Behavioural Brain Research*, 1984, *14*, 85–89.

Fozzard, H.A., & Schoenberg, M. Strength-duration curves in cardiac Purkinje fibres: Effect of liminal length and charge redistribution. *Journal of Physiology (London)*, 1972, *226*, 593–618.

Fritsch, G., & Hitzig, E. Ueber die elektrische Erregbarkeit des Grosshirns. *Archiv fuer Anatomie und Physiologie*, 1870, *37*, 300–332.

Fuller, J.H., & Schlag, J.D. Determination of antidromic excitation by the collision test: Problems of interpretation. *Brain Research*, 1976, *112*, 283–298.

Fuxe, K., Agnati, L.F., Kalia, M., Goldstein, M., Andersson, A., & Härfstrand, A. Dopaminergic systems in the brain and pituitary. In *The Dopaminergic System*, E. Flückiger, E.E. Müller & M.O. Thorner (Eds.). Berlin: Springer-Verlag, 1985. pp. 11–25.

Gallistel, C.R. Self-stimulation: The neurophysiology of reward and motivation. In *The Physiological Basis of Memory*, J.A. Deutsch (Ed.). New York: Academic Press, 1973. pp. 175–267.

Gallistel, C.R. Self-stimulation in the rat: Quantitative characteristics of the reward pathway. *Journal of Comparative and Physiological Psychology*, 1978, *92*, 977–998.

Gallistel, C.R. Subcortical stimulation for motivation and reinforcement. In *Electrical Stimulation Research Techniques*, M.M. Patterson and R.P. Kesner (Eds.). New York: Academic Press, 1981. pp. 141–171.

Gallistel, C.R. Self-stimulation. In *The Physiological Basis of Memory*, J.A. Deutsch (Ed.). New York: Academic Press, 1983. pp. 269–349.

Gallistel, C.R., Shizgal, P., & Yeomans, J.S. A portrait of the substrate for self-stimulation. *Physiological Review*, 1981, *88*, 228–273.

Geddes, L.A. A short history of the electrical stimulation of excitable tissue, including electrotherapeutic applications. *The Physiologist, Supp. 2*, 1984, 1–47.

Geddes, L.A., & Baker, L.E. The specific resistance of biological material—a compendium of data for the biomedical engineer and physiologist. *Medical and Biological Engineering*, 1967, *5*, 271–293.

Gerfen, C.R., & Sawchenko, P.E. An anterograde neuroanatomical tracing method that shows the detailed morphology of neurons, their axons and terminals—immunohistochemical localization of an axonally transported plant lectin Phaseolus-vulgaris leukoagglutinin (PHA-L). *Brain Research*, 1984, *290*, 219–238.

German, D.C., Dalsass, M., & Kiser, R.S. Electrophysiological examination of the ventral tegmental (A10) area in the rat. *Brain Research*, 1980, *181*, 191–197.

Girvin, J.P. A review of basic aspects concerning chronic cerebral stimulation. In *Cerebellar Stimulation in Man*, I.S. Cooper (Ed.) New York: Raven Press, 1978. pp. 1–12.

Girvin, J.P., Evans, J.R., Dobelle, W.H., Mladejovsky, M.G., Henderson, D.C., Abramov, I., Gordon, J., & Turkel, J. Electrical stimulation of human cortex: the effect of stimulus parameters on phosphene threshold. *Sensory Processes*, 1979, *3*, 66–81.

Glasstone, S. *Principles of Electrochemistry*. New York: Van Nostrand, 1946.

Gotch, F., & Burch, G.J. The electrical response of nerve to two stimuli. *Journal of Physiology (London)*, 1899, *24*, 410–426.

Grace, A.A., & Bunney, B.S. Intracellular and extracellular electrophysiology of nigral dopaminergic neurons—1. identification and characterization. *Neuroscience*, 1983, *10*, 301–315.

Grace, A.A., & Bunney, B.S. Opposing effects of striatonigral feedback pathways on midbrain dopamine cell activity. *Brain Research*, 1985, *333*, 271–284.

Graham, H.T. Supernormality, a modification of the recovery process in nerve. *American Journal of Physiology*, 1934, *110*, 225.

Grantyn, A., & Grantyn, R. Axonal patterns and sites of termination of cat superior colliculus neurons projecting in the tecto-bulbo-spinal tract. *Experimental Brain Research*, 1982, *46*, 243–256.

Gratton, A., & Wise, R.A. Brain stimulation reward in the lateral hypothalamic medial forebrain bundle: Mapping of boundaries and homogeneity. *Brain Research*, 1983, *274*, 25–30.

Gratton, A., & Wise, R.A. Hypothalamic reward mechanisms—Two first-stage fiber populations with a cholinergic component. *Science*, 1985, *227*, 545–548.

Gratton, A., & Wise, R.A. Comparisons of connectivity and conduction velocities for medial forebrain bundle fibers subserving stimulation-induced feeding and brain stimulation reward. *Brain Research*, 1988, *438*, 264–270.

Grillner, S., & Lund, S. The origin of a descending pathway with monosynaptic action on flexor motoneurons. *Acta Physiologica Scandinavica*, 1968, *74*, 274–284.

Guitton, D., & Mandl, G. Frontal 'oculomotor' area in alert cat. I. Eye movements and neck activity evoked by stimulation. *Brain Research*, 1978, *149*, 295–312.

Gustafsson, B., & Jankowska, E. Direct and indirect activation of nerve cells by electrical pulses applied extracellularly. *Journal of Physiology (London)*, 1976, *258*, 33–61.

Guyenet, P.G., & Aghajanian, G.K. Antidromic identification of dopaminergic and the other output neurons of the rat substantia nigra. *Brain Research*, 1978, *150*, 69–84.

Hall, R.D., & Lindholm, E.P. Organization of motor and somatosensory neocortex in the albino rat. *Brain Research*, 1974, *66*, 23–38.

Halgren, E. Mental phenomena induced by stimulation in the limbic system. *Human Neurobiology*, 1982, *1*, 251–260.

Hawkins, R.D., Roll, P.L., Puerto, A., & Yeomans, J.S. Refractory periods of neurons mediating stimulation-elicited eating and brain-stimulation reward: Interval scale measurement and tests of a model of integration. *Behavioral Neuroscience*, 1983, *97*, 416–432.

Hecht, S., Shlaer, S., & Pirenne, M.H. Energy, quanta and vision. *Journal of General Physiology*, 1942, *25*, 819–840.

Helmholtz, H.L.F. *Müller's Archiv der Anatomie und Physiologie*, 1850, 276–364.

Helmholtz, H. Über die Geschwindigkeit einiger Vorgänge in Muskeln und Nerven. *Bericht über die zur Bekanntmachung geeigneten Verhandlungen der König. Preussische Akademie der Wissenschaften zu Berlin*, 1854, 328–332. (cited in Gallistel, 1973).

Henneman, E., Somjen, G., & Carpenter, D.O. Functional significance of cell size in spinal motoneurons. *Journal of Neurophysiology*, 1965, *28*, 560–580.

Hentall, I.D. The membrane potential along an ideal axon in a radial electric field. *Brain Research*, 1985, *336*, 387–389.

Hentall, I.D., Zorman, G., Kansky, S., & Fields, H. An estimate of the minimum number of brain stem neurons required for inhibition of a flexion reflex. *Journal of Neurophysiology*, 1984, *5*, 978–985.

Hess, C.W., Mills, K.R., & Murray, N.M.F. Responses in small hand muscles from magnetic stimulation of the human brain. *Journal of Physiology*, 1987, *388*, 397–419.

Hess, C.W., Mills, K.R., & Murray, N.M.F. Magnetic stimulation of the human brain: The effects of voluntary muscle activity. *Journal of Physiology*, 1986, *378*, 37P.

Hess, W.R. *The Functional Organization of the Diencephalon*. New York: Greene & Stratton, 1957.

Hikosaka, O., & Wurtz, R.H. Modification of saccadic eye movements by GABA-related substances. I. Effect of muscimol and bicuculline in monkey superior colliculus. *Journal of Neurophysiology*, 1985a, *53*, 266–291.

Hikosaka, O., & Wurtz, R.H. Modification of saccadic eye movements by GABA-related substances. II. Effects of muscimol in monkey substantia nigra pars reticulata. *Journal of Neurophysiology*, 1985b, *53*, 292–308.

Hille, B. Excitability and ionic channels. In *Basic Neurochemistry*, G.J. Siegal, R.W. Albers, B.W. Agranoff, & R. Katzman (Eds.). Boston: Little Brown, 1981. pp. 95–106.

Hinsey, J.C., Ranson, S.W., & Dixon, H.H. Responses elicited by stimulation of the mesencephalic tegmentum in the cat. *Archives of Neurology and Psychiatry*, 1930, *24*, 966–977.

Hodgkin, A.L. The subthreshold potentials in a crustacean nerve fibre. *Proceedings of the Royal Society of Biology*, 1938, *126*, 87–121.

Hodgkin, A.L. Beginning—some reminiscences of my early life. *Annual Review of Physiology*, 1983, *45*, 1–16.

Hodgkin, A.L., & Rushton, W.A.H. The electrical constants of a crustacean nerve fibre. *Proceedings of the Royal Society (London)*, 1946, B133, 444–479.

Hodgkin, A.L., & Huxley, A.F. A quantitative description of membrane current and its application to conduction and excitation in nerve. *Journal of Physiology (London)*, 1952, *117*, 500–544.

Hu, J.W., & Coons, E.E. The neural refractory period of brain self-stimulation of reward: Effect of varying frequency. *Federation Proceedings*, 1975, *34*, 373.

Hubel, D. H., & Wiesel, T.N. Receptive fields, binocular interaction and functional architecture of cat's visual cortex. *Journal of Physiology (London)*, 1962, *160*, 106–154.

Huerta, M.F., & Harting, J.K. Tectal control of spinal cord activity: Neuroanatomical demonstration of pathways connecting the superior colliculus with the cervical spinal cord grey. In *Descending Pathways to the Spinal Cord*, H.G.J.M. Kuypers & G.F. Martin (Eds.). Amsterdam: Elsevier, 1982. pp. 293–328.

Hursch, J.B. Conduction velocity and diameter of nerve fibers. *American Journal of Physiology*, 1939, *127*, 131–139.

Iacono, R.P., & Nashold, B.S. Mental and behavioral effects of brain stem and hypothalamic stimulation in man. *Human Neurobiology*, 1982, *1*, 273–279.

Isaacson, R.L. Brain stimulation effects related to those of lesions. In *Electrical Stimulation Research Techniques*, M.M. Patterson & R.P. Kesner (Eds.). New York: Academic Press, 1981. pp. 205–220.

Jack, J.J.B., Noble, D., & Tsien, R.W. *Electric Current Flow in Excitable Cells*. London: Oxford University Press, 1975, 1983.

Jankowska, E., Padel, Y., & Tanaka, R. The mode of activation of pyramidal tract cells by intracortical stimulation. *Journal of Physiology (London)*, 1975, *249*, 617–636.

Katz, B. *Electrical Excitation of Nerve: a Review*. London: Oxford University Press, 1939.

Kennedy, C., Des Rosiers, M.H., Jehle, J.W., Reivich, M., Sharpe, F., & Sokoloff, L. Mapping of functional neural pathways by autoradiographic survey of local metabolic rate with [14C]deoxyglucose. *Science*, 1975, *187*, 850–852.

Kernell, D., & Wu, C.-P. Responses of the pyramidal tract to stimulation of the baboon's motor cortex. *Journal of Physiology (London)*, 1967, *191*, 653–672.

Kitai, S.T., Kocsis, J.D., Preston, R.J., & Sugimori, M. Monosynaptic inputs to caudate neurons identified by intracellular injection of horseradish peroxidase. *Brain Research*, 1976, *109*, 601–606.

Kocsis, J.D., Swadlow, H.A., Waxman, S.G., & Brill, M.H. Variation in conduction velocity during the relative refractory and supernormal periods: A mechanism for impulse entrainment in central axons. *Experimental Neurology*, 1979, *65*, 230–236.

Kofman, O. & Yeomans, J.S. Cholinergic antagonists in ventral tegmentum elevate thresholds for lateral hypothalamic and brainstem self-stimulation. *Physiology, Biochemistry and Behavior*, 1988, *31*, 547–559.

Krevs, P., Yeomans, J. & Buckenham, K. Refractory periods for hypothalamic self-stimulation are shortened by alpha-flupenthixol injections. *Society for Neuroscience Abstracts*, 1987 *13*, 1324.

Landgren, S., Phillips, C.G., & Porter, R. Cortical fields of origin of the monosynaptic pyramidal pathways to some alpha motoneurons of the baboon's hand and forearm. *Journal of Physiology (London)*, 1962, *161*, 112–125.

Leichnetz, G.R. The prefrontal cortico-oculomotor trajectories in the monkey: A possible explanation for the effects of stimulation/lesion experiments on eye movements. *Journal of the Neurological Sciences*, 1981, *49*, 387–396.

Lilly, J.C., Hughes, J.R., Alvord, E.C. Jr., & Galkin, T.W. Brief, noninjurious electrical waveform for stimulation of the brain. *Science*, 1955, *121*, 468–469.

Lipski, J. Antidromic activation of neurones as an analytic tool in the study of the central nervous system. *Journal of Neuroscience Methods*, 1981, *4*, 1–32.

Livingstone, M., & Hubel, D. Segregation of form, color, movement and depth: Anatomy, physiology and perception. *Science*, 1988, *240*, 740–749.

Lloyd, D.P.C. Facilitation and inhibition of spinal motorneurons. *Journal of Neurophysiology*, 1946, *9*, 421–438.

Lucas, K. *The Conduction of the Nervous Impulse.* Aberdeen: University Press, 1917(a).

Lucas, K. On summation of propagated disturbances in the claw of *Astacus* and on the double neural system of the adductor. *Journal of Physiology (London),* 1917(b), *51,* 1–35.

Maccabbee, P. J., Amassian, V.E., Cracco, R.Q., Cracco, J.B., & Anziska, B.J. Focal magnetic coil stimulation of human frontal cortex elicits speech related motor activity. *Society for Neuroscience Abstracts,* 1988, *14,* 159.

Macmillan, C. J., Simantirakis, P., & Shizgal, P. Self-stimulation of the lateral hypothalamus and ventrolateral tegmentum: Excitability characteristics of the directly stimulated substrates. *Physiology and Behavior,* 1985, *35,* 711–723.

Mark, V. H., & Ervin, F.R. *Violence and the Brain.* New York: Harper and Row, 1970.

Matthews, G.G. Neural substrate for brain stimulation reward in the rat: Cathodal and anodal strength-duration properties. *Journal of Comparative and Physiological Psychology,* 1977, *91,* 858–874.

Matthews, G. Strength-duration properties of single units driven by electrical stimulation of the lateral hypothalamus in rats. *Brain Research Bulletin,* 1978, *3,* 171–174.

McNeal, D.R. Two thousand years of electrical stimulation. In *Functional Electrical Stimulation,* F.T. Hambrecht & J.B. Reswick (Eds.). New York: Dekker, 1977. pp. 3–35.

Merton, P.A., & Morton, H.B. Stimulation of the cerebral cortex in the intact human subject. *Nature,* 1980, *285,* 227.

Miliaressis, E. Refractoriness of neurons subserving circling following stimulation of the median raphe region in the rat. *Physiology and Behavior,* 1981, *26,* 709–713.

Miliaressis, E., & Gratton, A. A chronic moveable non-rotating electrode for brain stimulation in the rat. *Physiology and Behavior,* 1981, *26,* 891–894.

Miliaressis, E., & Phillippe, L. A dual moveable electrode and its application to the behavioral version of the collision test. *Brain Research Bulletin,* 1983, *10,* 573–577.

Miliaressis, E., Rompre, P.-P., & Durivage, A. A psychophysical method for mapping behavioral substrates using a moveable electrode. *Brain Research Bulletin,* 1983, *8,* 693–701.

Mills, K.R., & Murray, N.M.F. Electrical stimulation over the human vertebral column: Which neural elements are excited? *Electroencephalography and Clinical Neurophysiology,* 1986, *63,* 582–589.

Milner, P.M., & Laferriere, A. Strength-duration characteristics of lateral hypothalamic and periaqueductal gray reward-path neurons. *Physiology and Behavior,* 1982, *29,* 857–863.

Milner, P.M., & Laferriere, A. Behavioral measurement of axonal thresholds. *Behavioural Brain Research,* 1986, *22,* 217–226.

Mountcastle, V.B. Modality and topographic properties of single neurons of cat's somatic sensory cortex. *Journal of Neurophysiology,* 1957, *20,* 408–434.

Mundl, W. A constant-current stimulator. *Physiology and Behavior,* 1980, *24,* 991–993.

Myklebust, J. B., Cusick, J.F., Sances, A., & Larson, S.J. *Neural Stimulation, Vols. I and II.* Boca Raton: CRC Press, 1985.

Neafsey, E. J., Bold, E. L., Haas, G., Hurley-Guis, K.M., Quirk, G., Sievert, C.F., & Terreberry, R.R. The organization of the rat motor cortex: A microstimulation mapping study. *Brain Research Reviews,* 1986, *11,* 77–96.

Neher, E., & Sakmann, B. Single channel currents recorded from membrane of denervated frog muscle fibres. *Nature,* 1976, *260,* 789–802.

Nieuwenhuys, R., Geeraedts, L.M.G., & Veening, J.G. The medial forebrain bundle of the rat. I. General introduction. *Journal of Comparative Neurology,* 1982, *206,* 49–81.

Noble, D., & Stein, R.B. The threshold conditions for initiation of action potentials by excitable cells. *Journal of Physiology* (London), 1966, *187,* 129–162.

Norman, M.F., & Gallistel, C.R. What can one learn from a strength-duration experiment? *Journal of Mathematical Physiology,* 1978, *18,* 1–27.

Noda, M., Ikeda, T., Kayano, T., Suzuki, H., Takeshima, H., et al. Existence of distinct sodium channel messenger RNAs in rat brain. *Nature,* 1986, *320,* 188–192.

Ojemann, G.A. Models of the brain organization for higher integrative functions derived with electrical stimulation techniques. *Human Neurobiology,* 1982, *1,* 243–249.

Olds, J., & Milner, P. Positive reinforcement produced by electrical stimulation of the septal area and other regions of the rat brain. *Journal of Comparative and Physiological Psychology,* 1954, *47,* 419–428.

Olds, M.E., & Fobes, J.L. The central basis of motivation: Intracranial self-stimulation studies. *Annual Review of Psychology,* 1981, *32,* 523–574.

Paintal, A.S. Conduction properties of normal peripheral mammalian axons. In *Physiology and Pathobiology of Axons,* S. Waxman (Ed.). New York: Raven Press, 1978. pp. 131–144.

Patton, H.D., & Amassian, V.E. Single- and multiple-unit analysis of cortical stage of pyramidal tract activation. *Journal of Neurophysiology,* 1954, *17,* 345–363.

Paxinos, G., & Watson, C. *The Rat Brain in Stereotaxic Coordinates.* Sydney: Academic Press, 1982.

Penfield, W., & Jasper, H.H. *Epilepsy and the Functional Anatomy of the Human Brain.* Boston: Little, Brown, 1954.

Peterson, B.W., Pitts, N.G., & Fukushima, K. Reticulospinal connections with limb and axial motoneurons. *Experimental Brain Research,* 1979, *36,* 1–20.

Phillips, A.G., & Fibiger, H.C. The role of dopamine in maintaining intracranial self-stimulation in the ventral tegmentum, nucleus accumbens and medial prefrontal cortex. *Canadian Journal of Psychology,* 1978, *32,* 58–66.

Phillips, C.G., & Porter, R. *Corticospinal Neurones.* London: Academic Press, 1977.

Pudenz, R. H., Agnew, W.F., & Bullara, L.A. Effects of electrical stimulation of brain: Light- and electron-microscope studies. *Brain, Behavior and Evolution,* 1977, *14,* 103–125.

Pudenz, R.H., Bullara, L.A., & Talalla, A. Electrical stimulation of the brain. I. Electrodes and electrode arrays. *Surgical Neurology,* 1975, *4,* 37–42.

Pycock, C. J. Turning behavior in animals. *Neuroscience,* 1980, *5,* 461–516.

Ranck, J.B. Jr. Which elements are excited in electrical stimulation of mammalian central nervous system: A review. *Brain Research,* 1975, *98,* 417–440.

Ranck, J.B. Jr. Extracellular stimulation. In *Electrical Stimulation Research Techniques,* M.M. Patterson & R.P. Kesner (Eds.). New York: Academic Press, 1981. pp. 1–36.

Raymond, S.A., & Lettvin, J.Y. Aftereffects of activity in peripheral axons as a clue to nervous coding. In *Physiology and Pathobiology of Axons,* S.G. Waxman (Ed.). New York: Raven Press, 1978. pp. 203–225.

Redgrave, P., Mitchell, I.J., & Dean, P. Descending projections from the superior colliculus in rat: A study using orthograde transport of wheatgerm-agglutinin conjugated horseradish peroxidase. *Experimental Brain Research,* 1987, *198,* 147–167.

Redgrave, P., Odekunle, A., & Dean, P. Tectal cells of origin of predorsal bundle in rat: Location and segregation from ipsilateral descending pathway. *Experimental Brain Research,* 1986, *63,* 279–293.

Richardson, T.L., Miller, J.J., & McLennan, H. Mechanisms of excitation and inhibition in the nigrostriatal system. *Brain Research,* 1977, *127,* 219–234.

Roberts, W. J., & Smith, D.O. Analysis of threshold currents during microstimulation of fibres in the spinal cord. *Acta Physiologica Scandinavica,* 1973, *89,* 384–394.

Robinson, D.A., & Fuchs, A.F. Eye movements evoked by stimulation of frontal eye fields. *Journal of Neurophysiology,* 1969, *32,* 637–648.

Rolls, E.T. Involvement of brainstem units in medial forebrain bundle self-stimulation. *Physiology and Behavior,* 1971, *7,* 297–310.

Rolls, E.T. The neural basis of brain-stimulation reward. *Progress in Neurobiology,* 1974, *3,* 71–160.

Rompre, P.-P., Miliaressis, E. A comparison of the excitability cycles of the hypothalamic fibers involved in self-stimulation and exploration. *Physiology and Behavior,* 1980, *24,* 995–998.

Rompre, P.-P., & Miliaressis, E. Behavioral determination of refractory periods of the brain stem substrates of self-stimulation. *Behavioural Brain Research,* 1987, *23,* 205–219.

Rompre, P.-P., & Shizgal, P. Electrophysiological characteristics of neurons in forebrain regions implicated in self-stimulation of the medial forebrain bundle in the rat. *Brain Research,* 1986, *364,* 338–349.

Rose, P.K., & Abrahams, V.C. Tectospinal and tectoreticular cells: Their distribution and afferent connections. *Canadian Journal of Physiology and Pharmacology,* 1978, *56,* 650–658.

Ruch, T.C., Patton, H.D., Woodbury, J.W., & Towe, A.L. *Neurophysiology.* Philadelphia: W.B. Saunders, 1965.

Rushton, W.A.H. Effect upon the threshold for nervous activation of the length of nerve exposed and the angle between current and nerve. *Journal of Physiology (London),* 1927, *63,* 357–377.

Rushton, W.A.H. The site of excitation in the nerve trunk of the frog. *Journal of Physiology,* 1949, *109,* 314–326.

Schenk, S., & Shizgal, P. The substrates for lateral hypothalamic and medial pre-frontal cortex self-stimulation have different refractory periods and show poor spatial summation. *Physiology and Behavior,* 1982, *28,* 133–138.

Schiller, P.H. The effects of superior colliculus ablations on saccades elicited by cortical stimulation. *Brain Research,* 1977, *122,* 154–156.

Schlag, J. Electrophysiological mapping techniques. In *Neuroanatomical Research Techniques,* R.F. Thompson (Ed.). New York: Academic Press, 1978.

Sheer, D.E. (Ed.). *Electrical Stimulation of the Brain.* Austin: University of Texas Press, 1961.

Sherrington, C.S. *The Integrative Action of the Nervous System.* New Haven: Yale University Press, 1906.

Shizgal, P., Bielajew, C., Corbett, D., Skelton, R., & Yeomans, J.S. Behavioral methods for inferring anatomical linkage between rewarding brain stimulation sites. *Journal of Comparative and Physiological Psychology,* 1980, *94,* 227–237.

Shizgal, P., Howlett, S., & Corbett, D. Behavioral inference of current–distance relationships in rewarding electrical stimulation of the rat hypothalamus. Poster presented at Canadian Psychological Association meeting, 1979.

Shizgal, P., & Murray, B. Neuronal basis of intracranial self-stimulation. In *The Neu-ropharmacological Basis of Reward,* J.M. Liebman and S.J. Cooper (Eds.). London: Oxford Univ. Press, 1989, 106–163.

Shizgal, P. & Schindler, D.C. A model of spatial and temporal integration in the substrate for brain stimulation reward. In preparation.

Silva, L.R., Vogel, J.A., & Corbett, D. Frontal cortex self-stimulation: Evidence for independent substrates within areas 32 and 24. *Society for Neuroscience Abstracts,* 1982, *8*, 625.

Sinnamon, H.M., & Galer, B.S. Head movements elicited by stimulation of the anteromedial cortex of the rat. *Physiology and Behavior,* 1984, *33*, 185–190.

Sinnamon, H.M. Forelimb and hindlimb stepping by the anesthetized rat elicited by electrical stimulation of the diencephalon and mesencephalon. *Physiology and Behavior,* 1984, *33*, 201–208.

Smith, N.S., & Coons, E.E. Temporal summation and refractoriness in hypothalamic reward neurons as measured by self-stimulation behavior. *Science,* 1970, *169*, 782–785.

Stein, B.E. Multimodal representation in the superior colliculus and optic tectum. In *Comparative Neurology of the Optic Tectum,* H. Vanegas (Ed.). New York: Plenum Press, 1984. pp. 819–841.

Stein, L. Norepinephrine reward pathways. Role in self-stimulation, memory consolidation, and schizophrenia. *Nebraska Symposium on Motivation,* 1975, *22*, 113–159.

Stellar, J., & Stellar, E. *Biology of Motivation and Reward.* New York: Springer-Verlag, 1986.

Stoney, S.D., Jr., Thompson, W.D., & Asanuma, H. Excitation of pyramidal tract cells by intracortical microstimulation: Effective extent of stimulating current. *Journal of Neurophysiology,* 1968, *31*, 659–669.

Swadlow, H.A. Impulse conduction in the mammalian brain: Physiological properties of individual axons monitored for several months. *Science,* 1982, *218*, 911–913.

Swadlow, H.A., & Waxman, S.G. Activity-dependent variations in the conduction properties of central axons. In *Physiology and Pathobiology of Axons,* S. Waxman, (Ed). New York: Raven Press, 1978. pp. 191–202.

Swadlow, H.A., Kocsis, J.D., & Waxman, S.G. Modulation of impulse conduction along the axonal tree. *Annual Review of Biophysics and Bioengineering,* 1980, *9*, 143–179.

Szabo, I. Path neuron system of medial forebrain bundle as a possible substrate for hypothalamic self-stimulation. *Physiology and Behavior,* 1973, *10*, 315–328.

Szabo, I. & Milner, P.M. Intracranial self-stimulation in the rat: Cable properties of the depolarized membrane. *Acta Physiologica Academiae Scientiarum Hungaricae,* 1973, *43*, 65–70.

Szabo, F., Nad, E., & Szabo, C. Pole reversals and hypothalamic self-stimulation: Ascending spread of reward excitation. *Physiology and Behavior,* 1972, *9*, 147–150.

Tasaki, I. Das Schwellenabsinken bei Reizung einer Nervenfaser mit kurzen Strömstossen. *Pflügers Archiv,* 1942, *245*, 665–679.

Tasaki, I. Conduction of the nerve impulse. In *Handbook of Physiology: Volume 1, Neurophysiology,* J. Field (Ed.). Washington: American Physiological Society, 1959. pp. 75–121.

Tasker, R.R., Organ, L.W., & Hawrylyshyn, P. *The Thalamus and Midbrain of Man: A Physiological Atlas using Electrical Stimulation.* Springfield, Ill.: Thomas, 1982.

Tehovnik, E.J., & Yeomans, J.S. Circling elicited from the anteromedial cortex and medial pons: Refractory periods and summation. *Brain Research,* 1987, *407,* 240–252.

Tehovnik, E.J., & Yeomans, J.S. Two converging brainstem pathways mediating circling behavior. *Brain Research,* 1986, *385,* 329–342.

Tehovnik, E.J., & Yeomans, J.S. Contraversive circling elicited from the internal capsule and substantia nigra: Evidence for continuous axons mediating circling. *Brain Research,* 1988, *441,* 269–280.

Towe, A.L. Motor cortex and the pyramidal system. In *Efferent Organization and Integration of Behavior,* J.D. Mason, (Ed.). New York: Academic Press, 1973.

Vallbo, A.B., Olsson, K.A., Westberg, K.-G., & Clark, F.J. Microstimulation of single tactile afferents from the human hand. *Brain,* 1984, *107,* 727–749.

Valenstein, E.S. *Brain Control: A Critical Examination of Brain Stimulation and Psychosurgery.* New York: Wiley, 1973.

Valenstein, E.S., Cox, V.C., & Kakolewski, J.W. A reexamination of the role of the hypothalamus in motivation. *Psychological Review,* 1970, *77,* 16–31.

Velley, L. The role of intrinsic neurons in lateral hypothalamic self-stimulation. *Behavioural Brain Research,* 1986, *22,* 141–152.

Wagman, I.H. Eye movements induced by electrical stimulation of cerebrum in monkeys and their relationship to body movements. In *The Oculomotor System,* M.B. Bender (Ed.). New York: Harper and Row, 1964. pp. 17–39.

Wall, P.D., McCulloch, W.S., Lettvin, J.Y., & Pitts, W.H. The terminal arborization of the cat's pyramidal tract determined by a new technique. *Yale Journal of Biological Medicine,* 1956, *28,* 457–464.

Ward, H.P. Stimulus factors in septal self-stimulation. *American Journal of Physiology,* 1959, *196,* 774–782.

Waxman, S.G. (Ed.) *Physiology and Pathobiology of Axons.* New York: Raven Press, 1978.

Weiss, G. Sur la possibilité de rendre comparables entre eux les appareils servant a l'excitation. *Archivi Italiani de Biologia,* 1901, *35,* 413–446.

West, D.C., & Wolstencroft, J.H. Strength-duration characteristics of myelinated and non-myelinated bulbospinal axons in the cat spinal cord. *Journal of Physiology (London),* 1983, *337,* 37–50.

White, N. Strength-duration analysis of the organization of reinforcement pathways in the medial forebrain bundle of rats. *Brain Research,* 1976, *110,* 575–591.

Wise, R.A. Catecholamine theories of reward: A critical review. *Brain Research,* 1978, *22,* 535–542.

Wise, R.A. Action of drugs of abuse on brain reward systems. *Pharmacology, Biochemistry and Behavior,* 1981, *13,* Suppl. (1), 213–223.

Wolf, G. Elementary histology for neuropsychologists. In *Methods in Psychobiology, Volume 1,* R.D. Myers (Ed.). New York: Academic Press, 1971. pp. 281–299.

Wong-Riley, M. Changes in the visual system of monocularly sutured or enucleated cats demonstrable with cytochrome oxidase histochemistry. *Brain Research,* 1979, *171,* 11–28.

Woolsey, C.N. Organization of somatic sensory and motor areas of the cerebral cortex. In *Biological and Biochemical Bases of Behavior,* H.F. Harlow & C.N. Woolsey (Eds.). Madison, Wisc.: University of Wisconsin Press, 1958. pp. 63–81.

Yeomans, J.S. Quantitative measurement of neural post-stimulation excitability with behavioral methods. *Physiology and Behavior,* 1975, *15,* 593–602.

Yeomans, J.S. Absolute refractory periods of self-stimulation neurons. *Physiology and Behavior,* 1979, *22,* 911–919.

Yeomans, J.S. The cells and axons mediating medial forebrain bundle reward. In, *The Neural Basis of Feeding and Reward*, B.G. Hoebel & D. Novin, (Eds.). Brunswick, Me.: Haer Institute, 1982. pp. 405–417.

Yeomans, J.S. Mechanisms of brain-stimulation reward. *Progress in Psychobiology and Physiological Psychology, Volume 13*, A.N. Epstein & A. Morrison (Eds.). Sarasota: Academic Press, 1988. pp. 227–266.

Yeomans, J.S. & Buckenham, K. Electrically-evoked turning: Asymmetric and symmetric collision between anteromedial cortex and striatum. *Society for Neuroscience Abstracts*, 1988, *14*, 956.

Yeomans, J.S., & Davis, J.K. Behavioral measurement of post-stimulation excitability of neurons mediating self-stimulation by varying the voltage of paired pulses. *Behavioral Biology*, 1975, *15*, 435–447.

Yeomans, J.S., Rosen, J., Barbeau, J., & Davis, M. Double pulse stimulation of startle-like responses in rats: Refractory periods and temporal summation. *Brain Research*, 1989, *486*, 547–559.

Yeomans, J.S., Gallistel, C.R., & Reivich M. Autoradiographic mapping of brain regions activated during self-stimulation using [14] C-2deoxyglucose. *Society for Neuroscience Abstracts*, 1978, *4*, 230.

Yeomans, J.S., Kofman, O., & McFarlane, V. Cholinergic involvement in lateral hypothalamic self stimulation. *Brain Research*, 1985, *329*, 19–26.

Yeomans, J.S., Kofman, O., & McFarlane, V. Cholinergic involvement in hypothalamic and midbrain rewarding brain stimulation. In *Biological Determinants of Reinforcement*, R.M. Church, M.L. Commons, J.R. Stellar, & A.R. Wagner (Eds.). Hillsdale, N.J.: Lawrence Erlbaum, 1988. pp. 87–102.

Yeomans, J.S., & Linney, L. Brainstem axons mediating circling: Behavioral measurement of conduction velocity distributions. *Behavioural Brain Research*, 1985, *15*, 121–135.

Yeomans, J.S., Maidment, N., & Bunney, B.S. Excitability properties of medial forebrain bundle axons of A9 and A10 dopamine cells. *Brain Research*, 1988, *450*, 86–93.

Yeomans, J.S., Matthews, G.G., Hawkins, R.D., Bellman, K., & Doppelt, H. Characterization of self-stimulation neurons by their local potential summation properties. *Physiology and Behavior*, 1979, *22*, 921–929.

Yeomans, J.S., Mercouris, N., & Ellard C. Refractory period estimates are lengthened by reducing electrode tip exposure or increasing current. *Behavioral Neuroscience*, 1985, *99*, 913–928.

Yeomans, J.S., Pearce, R., Wen, D., & Hawkins, R.D. Mapping midbrain sites for circling using current-frequency trade-off data. *Physiology and Behavior*, 1984, *32*, 287–294.

Yeomans, J.S., Prior, P., & Bateman, F. Behavioral estimation of the current–distance relationships of neurons mediating circling elicited by midbrain stimulation. *Brain Research*, 1986, *372*, 95–106.

Yeomans, J.S., & Tehovnik, E.J. Turning responses evoked by stimulation of visuomotor pathways. *Brain Research Reviews*, 1988, *13*, 235–259.

Index

35. M